Dear Reader,

Thank you so much for picking up The Glow Bar: Hydration Rituals for Women Who Don't Do Water. You are officially my kind of person.

Let's be honest... I write a lot of books. Between spicy fantasy sagas (Divine Submission), chaotic historical adventures (The MirrorVerse and The Realmsverse), and wildly unhinged characters who keep hijacking my plots, staying hydrated is essential.

But here's the problem: plain water? Tasteless. Emotionless. Utterly uninspiring. It's the literary equivalent of a soggy rice cake.

So, instead of sipping sadness, I started crafting beautiful, delicious drinks that spark joy and keep the creative flow flowing. These recipes are a mix of wellness, whimsy, and a little rebellion against boring hydration.

I hope you enjoy every sip as much as I do, whether you're reading, writing, relaxing, or simply refusing to drink another glass of disappointment.

Cheers to glowing from the inside out,
Holly Symons

The Glow Bar Shopping List

Before you sip your first glow-up in a glass, let's talk tools. You don't need a five-star kitchen or a mixology degree, just a few basic appliances and containers. I've included everything I personally use, plus a few optional goodies if you're the kind of hydration diva who likes your drinks on the go, spill-proof, and served with a little sass. Because let's face it: some of us are clumsy (me), and lids are lifesavers. But honestly? Use whatever you have and make it fabulous.

Must-Haves:
- Juicer
- Cold Brew Glass Coffee Maker / Iced Tea Maker
- Blender
- Coffee Maker (if using fresh ground coffee)
- Kettle (for boiling water for teas, instant coffee, hot chocolate)
- Ice Tray
- 1L Heatproof Glass Drink Bottles with Leak-Proof Lids (as many as you need)
- Clear Juice Containers
- Measuring spoons (for syrups, coffee, and hot chocolate scooping)

Optional Goodies:

- Coffee Mug with Lid / Travel Mug (Leak-Proof, Stainless Steel, Insulated Tumbler)
- Cold Drink Tumbler
- Glass Cups with Lids and Straws (Mason Jar Style for Iced Coffee, Smoothies, Long Drinks)
- Drink Bottles with Leak-Proof Stainless-Steel Lids (Clear Juice Containers)

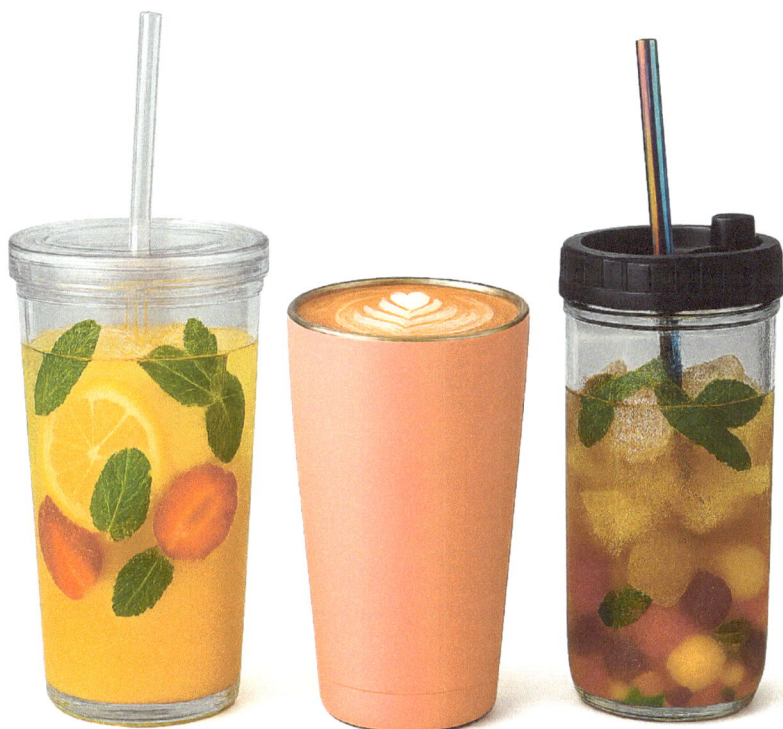

Juice Recipes _____ 2

   Sunrise Squeeze _____ 4

   Island Drift _____ 8

   Seafoam Glow_____ 10

   Ocean Cleanse _____ 12

   Coastal Crush _____ 14

   Citrus Siren _____ 16

   Sunset Kiss _____ 18

   Wicked Wave_____ 20

   Crimson Current _____ 22

   Lifeguard Elixir _____ 24

Glow Bar Boba Teas _____ 27

   Double Strawberry Green _____ 29

   Peach Green Tea_____ 31

   Grapefruit Green Tea_____ 33

   Passionfruit Green Tea _____ 35

   Lychee Oolong & Aloe_____ 37

   Mango Oolong _____ 39

Smoothies _____ 42

   Peach Yoghurt Smoothie _____ 43

   Mango Smoothie _____ 45

Mixed Berry Smoothie _____ 47

Blueberry Smoothie _____ 49

Frappes _____ 52

Mango Frappe _____ 54

Mixed Berry Frappe _____ 56

Blueberry Frappe _____ 58

Watermelon Frappe _____ 60

Caramel Frappe Milk_____ 62

Strawberry Frappe Milk _____ 64

Vanilla Frappe Milk _____ 66

Hazelnut Frappe Milk _____ 68

Mocha Frappe Milk _____ 70

*Glow Bar Cocktails*_____ 72

French Kiss _____ 74

Dunk Bunny Cocktail _____ 76

Sunset Sangria _____ 78

Pineapple Basil Mojito _____ 80

Rose & Lychee Sparkler _____ 82

Citrus Crown Cooler _____ 84

Mocktail Margarita _____ 86

Lavender Lemonade Spritz_____ 88

Amaretto Aloha _____ 90

.

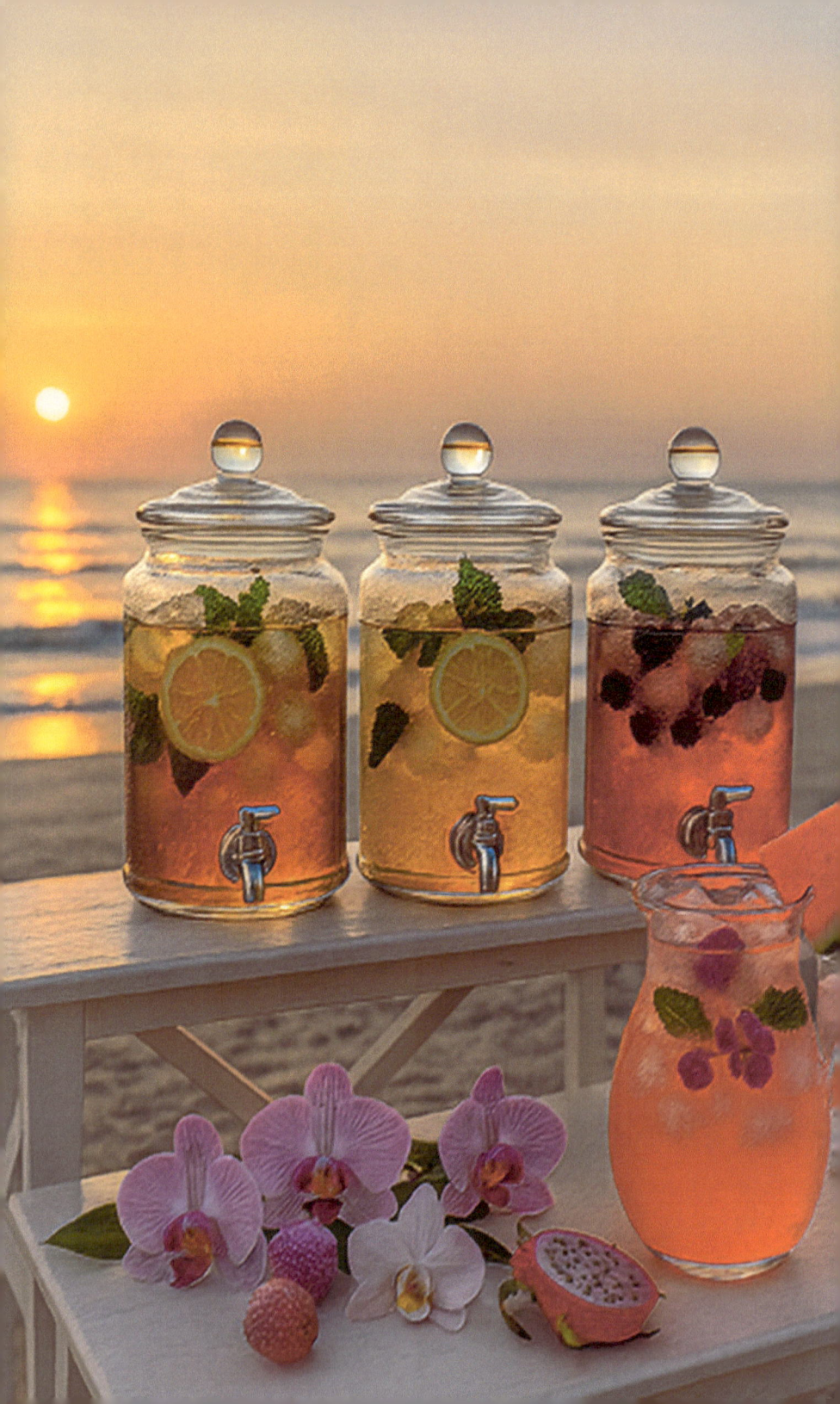

Juice Recipes

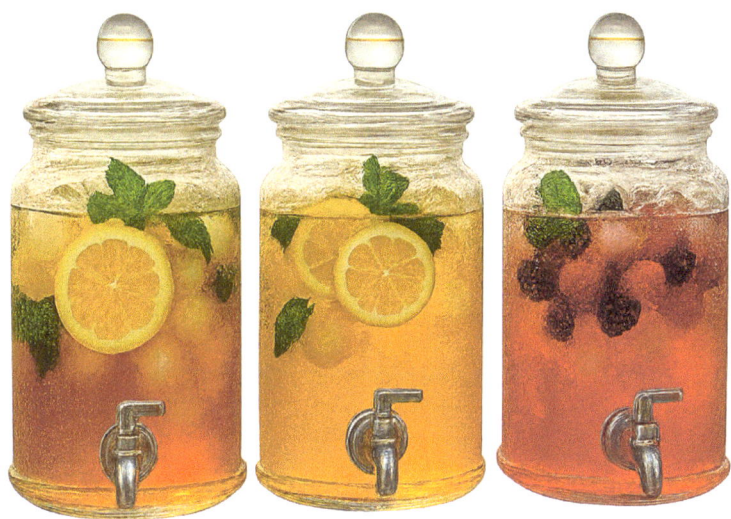

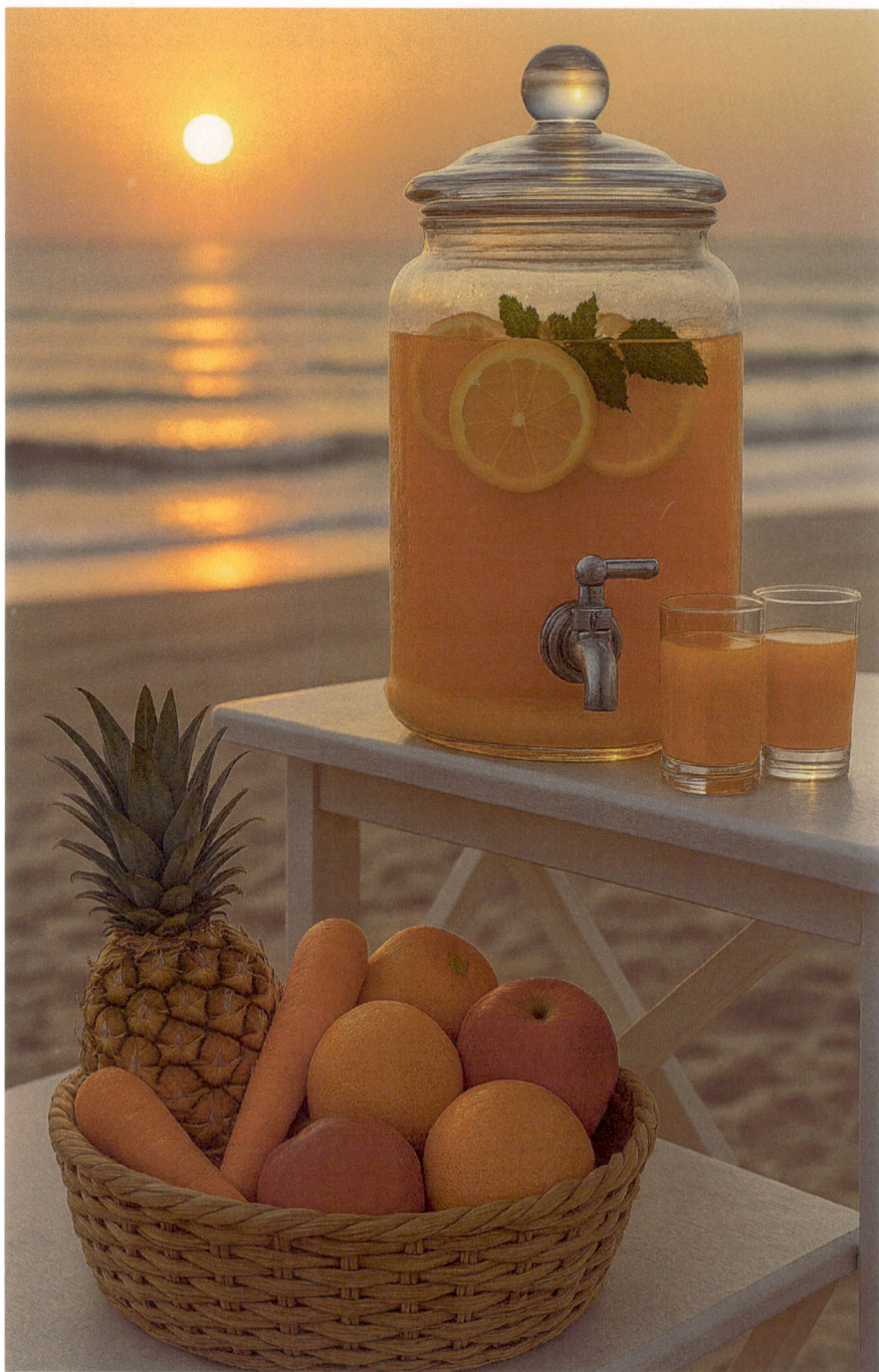

Sunrise Squeeze

Ingredients:

- 1 large orange
- 1 medium carrot
- 1 small apple (sweet variety)
- 1 generous slice of pineapple

Method:

Use a cold press juicer to gently extract the goodness from each ingredient, starting with the carrot and ending with the pineapple for a smooth, balanced blend.

Storage:

Pour into a 1L glass bottle with a leak-proof lid. This juice will keep its sunny charm for 2 to 3 days when stored in the fridge.

To Serve:

Pour over ice into a boba teacup with a wide straw because hydration is way more fun when it feels like a treat. Add a sprig of mint or an edible flower if you're feeling fancy.

*Sip and glow like you just watched the sunrise from a private beach.

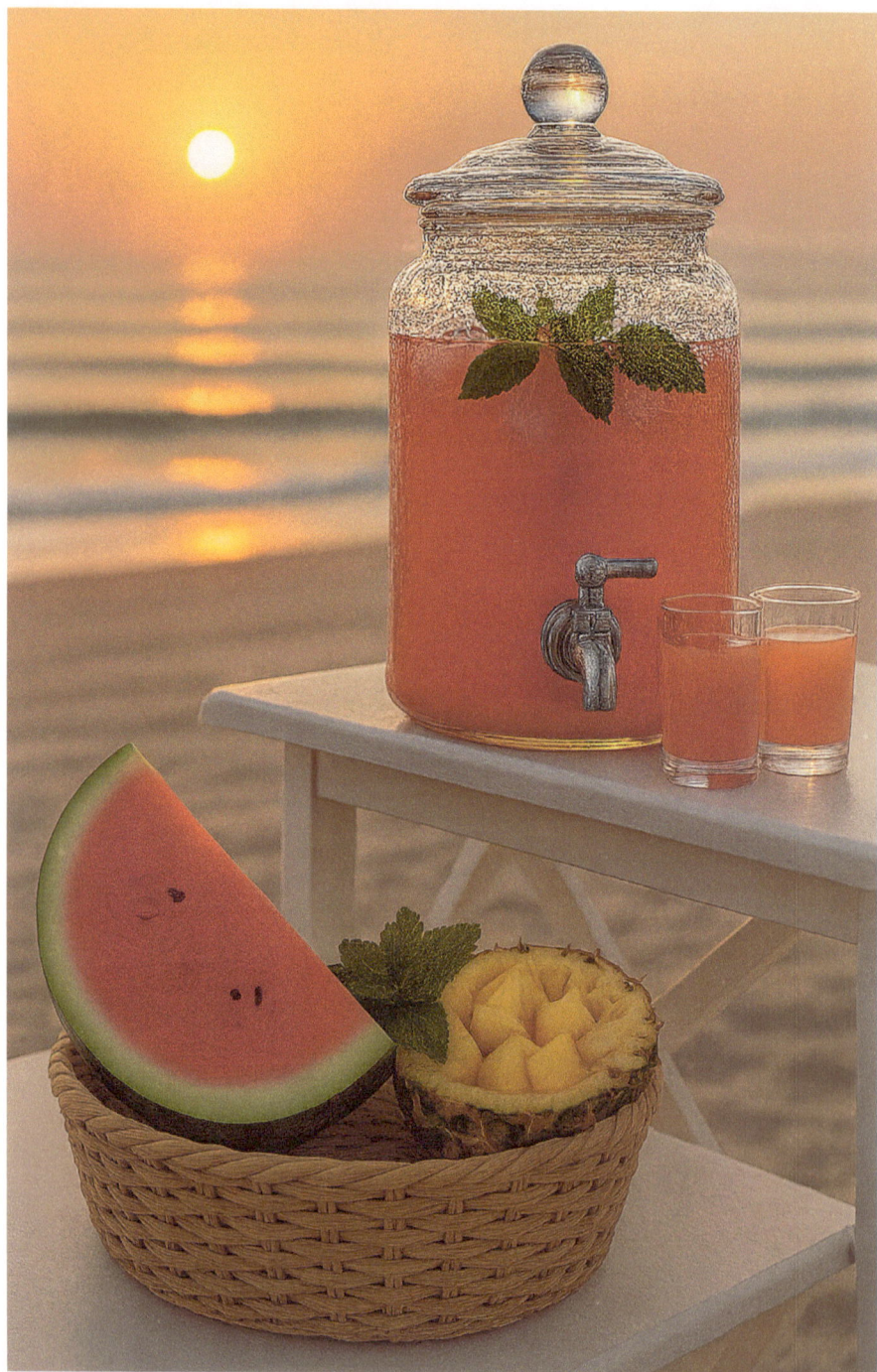

Tidebreaker Pink

Ingredients:

- 2 cups cubed watermelon (seedless if possible)
- 1 handful of fresh mint leaves
- 1 cup pineapple chunks

Method:

Feed all ingredients through a cold press juicer, starting with the pineapple to create a juicy base, then add the watermelon and mint. Press the mint between the fruits for best extraction.

Storage:

Store in a 1L clear glass bottle with a leak-proof lid and refrigerate. Best enjoyed within 2 to 3 days while it's fresh, fruity, and full of beachy vibes.

To Serve:

Serve chilled in a boba teacup with plenty of ice. Garnish with a small mint sprig or a tiny wedge of pineapple on the rim for that tropical vacation energy.

* Drink this one under a palm tree, real or imagined.

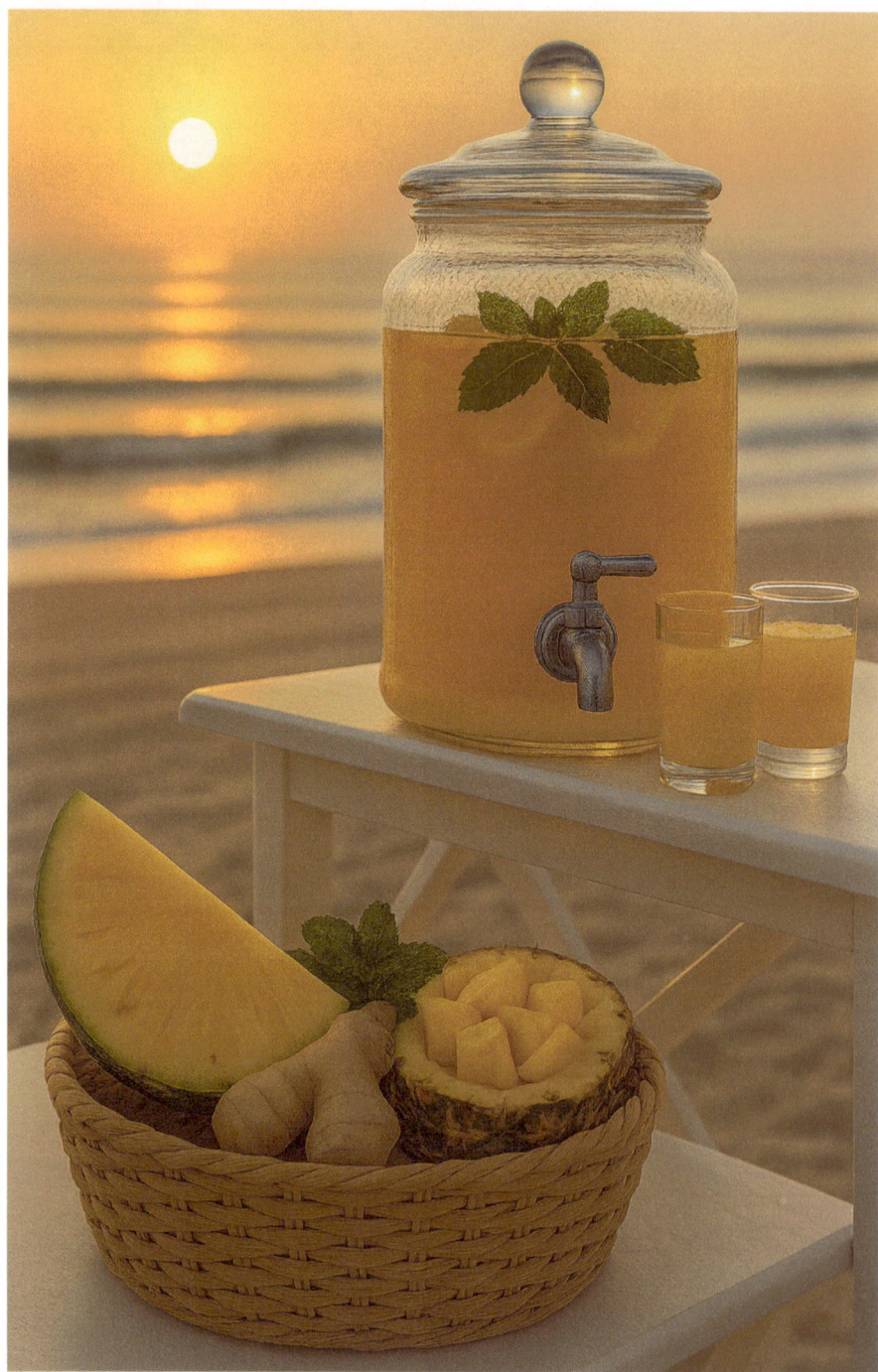

Island Drift

Ingredients:

- 1 cup pineapple chunks
- 1 small knob of fresh ginger (about 1 inch, peeled)
- 1 handful fresh mint leaves
- 1 ripe pear, chopped

Method:

Cold press each ingredient slowly, starting with the pineapple and ending with the mint for a bold finish. Feed the mint between the pear and pineapple for maximum juice and minimal mess.

Storage:

Transfer your tropical tonic into a 1L glass juice container with a tight-fitting lid. Keep chilled and sip within 2 to 3 days to enjoy peak flavour and island energy.

To Serve:

Pour over crushed ice in a tall smoothie glass or tumbler. Garnish with a pineapple leaf or slice of pear. Add a reusable straw, close your eyes, and you're drifting off to your favourite beach.

*Spicy. Sweet. Breezy. Just like your dream holiday.

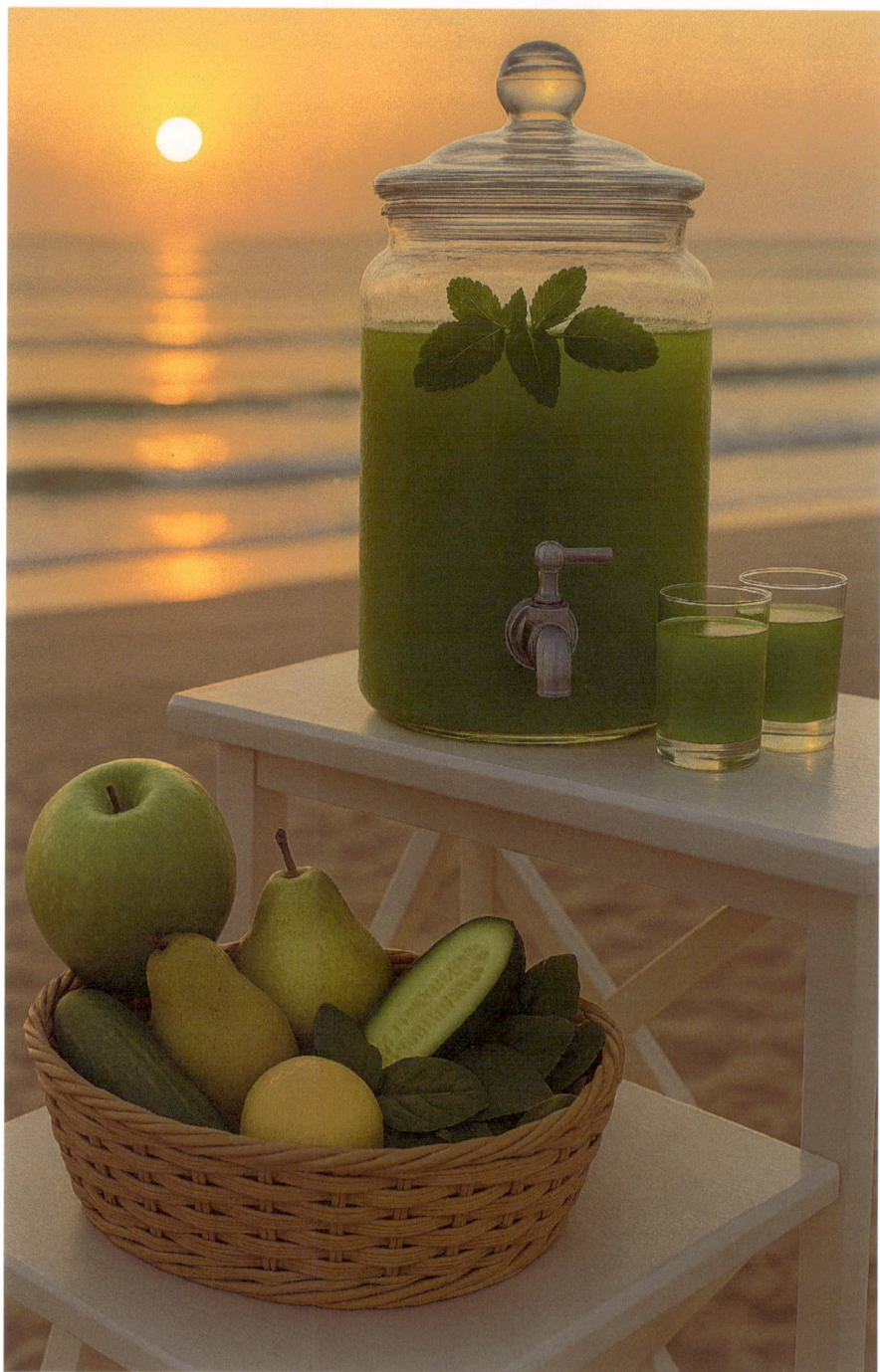

Seafoam Glow

Ingredients:

- 1 green apple
- 1 ripe pear
- 1/2 cucumber (peeled if waxed)
- 1 handful of baby spinach
- 1/2 lemon (peeled, seeds removed)

Method:

Cold-press all ingredients, starting with the spinach and lemon to help the juicer handle the softer items, then follow with the crisp cucumber, pear, and apple. The lemon brightens the entire blend with a refreshing kick.

Storage:

Store your glow potion in a leak-proof glass bottle in the fridge. It stays fresh and radiant for up to 3 days, but let's be honest, you'll drink it way before then.

To Serve:

Serve chilled in a clear glass with a slice of lemon or cucumber on the rim. Bonus points for sipping barefoot with sea breeze energy.

*Refreshing, light, and hydrating like a salty kiss from the sea.

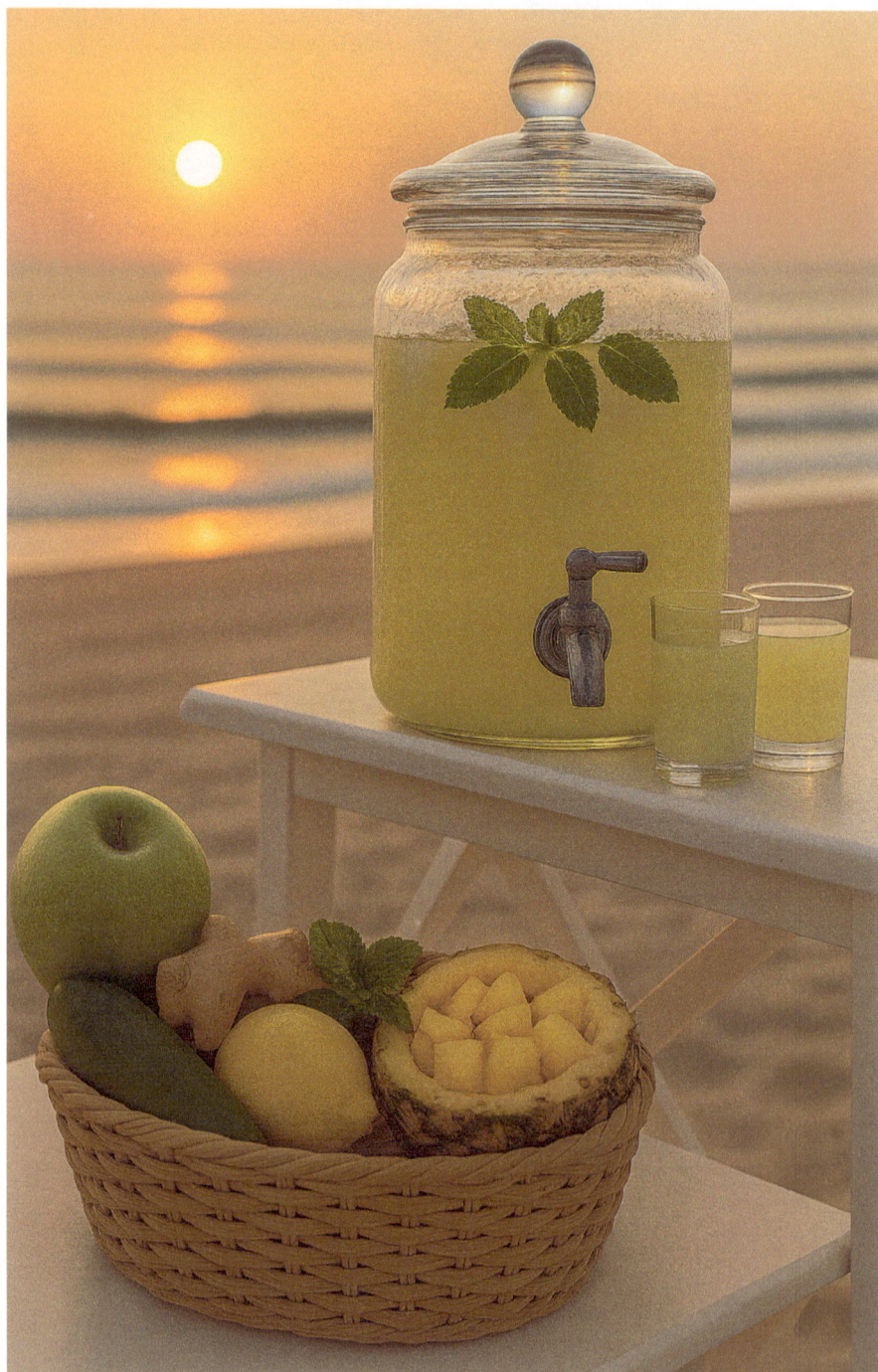

Ocean Cleanse

Ingredients:

- 1 green apple
- 1/2 cucumber (peeled if waxed)
- 1 handful of baby spinach
- 1 small knob fresh ginger (about 1 inch, peeled)
- 1 cup pineapple chunks

Method:

Begin with the leafy spinach and ginger, then follow with cucumber, apple, and pineapple. Use a cold press juicer to slowly extract every drop of vitamin-packed glow from these hydrating ingredients.

Storage:

Pour into a 1L glass juice bottle and store in the fridge. This one tastes best icy cold and lasts 2–3 days without losing its wave of freshness.

To Serve:

Serve over ice in a mason jar or spa tumbler with a sprig of mint or a cucumber ribbon. Put on ocean sounds and pretend you're detoxing from a luxury retreat.

*Light, cleansing, and quietly powerful just like the tide.

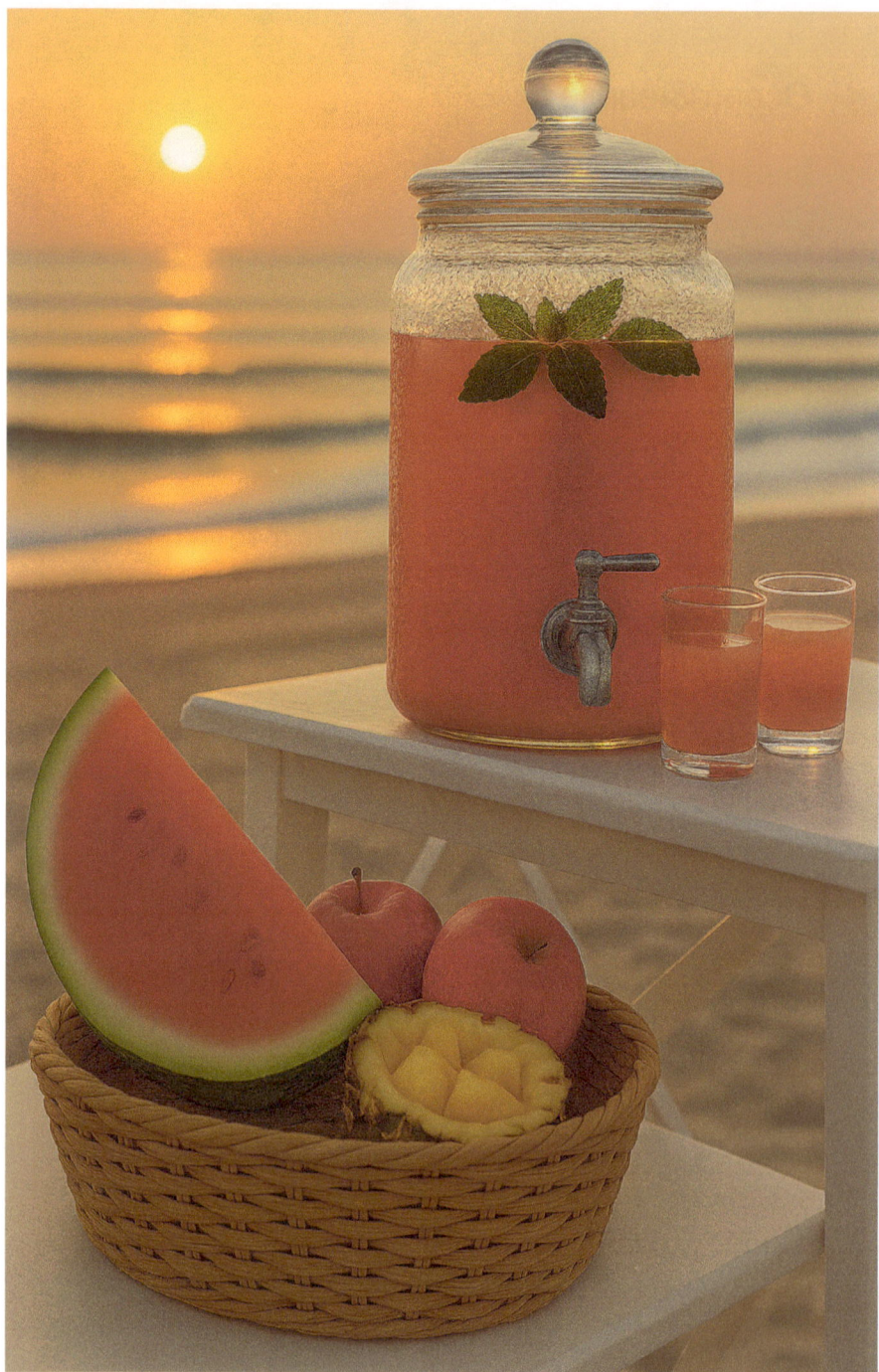

Coastal Crush

Ingredients:

- 2 cups cubed watermelon (seedless)
- 1 sweet red apple
- 1 cup pineapple chunks

Method:

Juice the pineapple and apple first, then follow with the watermelon to balance the sweetness and add a juicy finish. Use a cold press juicer to preserve the fresh, sun-drenched flavour.

Storage:

Store in a glass juice bottle with a leak-proof lid. This juice is best enjoyed within 48 hours while the watermelon's tropical magic is still popping.

To Serve:

Pour over crushed ice in a tall glass. Add a wedge of watermelon or a pineapple leaf for garnish. Drink with sandy feet and salty hair, if possible.

*Sweet, chill, and ready to party like a summer fling in a cup.

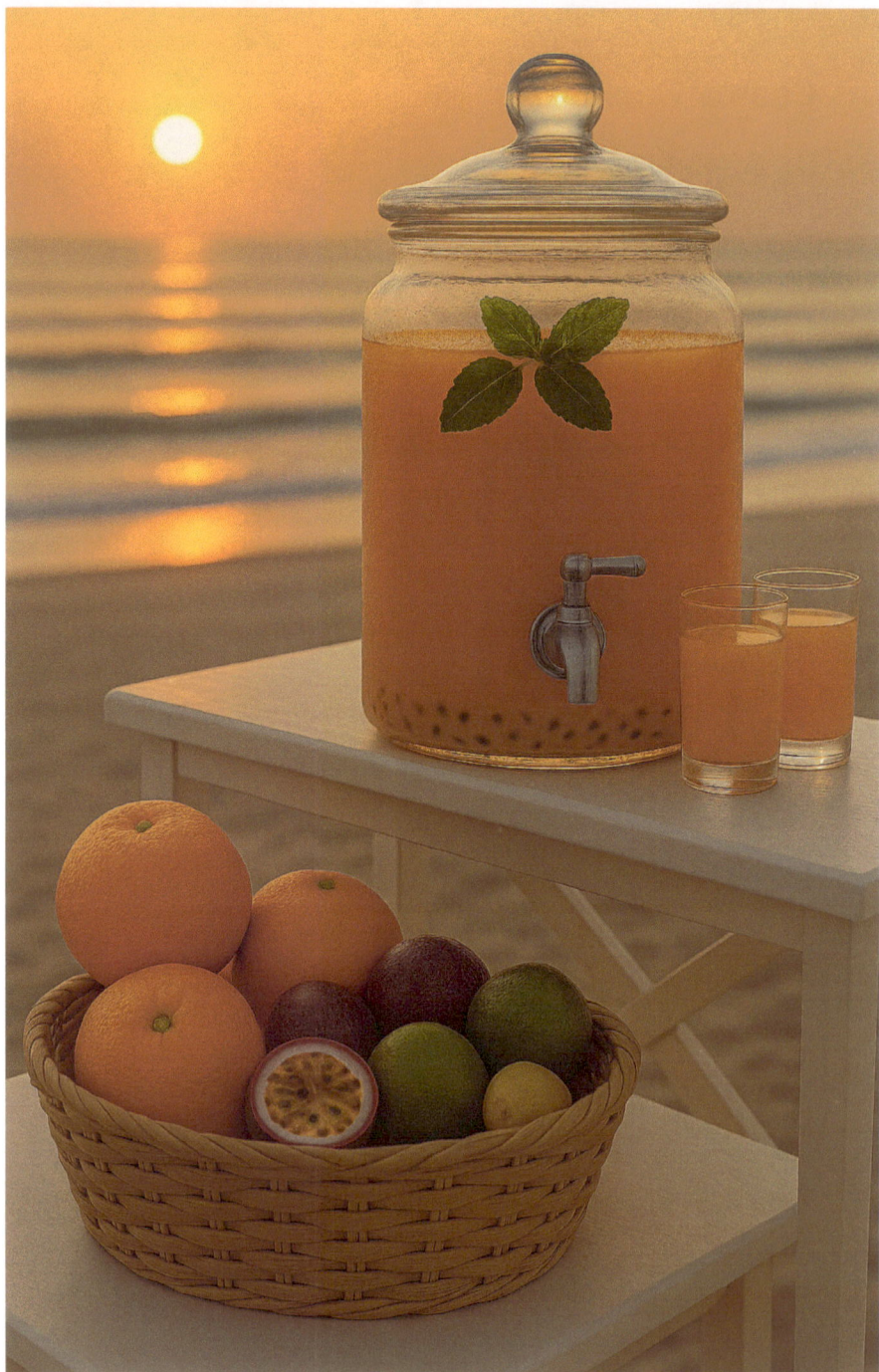

Citrus Siren

Ingredients:

- 2 large oranges (peeled)
- 2 passionfruit (scooped pulp only)
- 1/2 lime (peeled)

Method:

Cold-press the orange and lime first for a smooth citrus base. Then stir in the passionfruit pulp by hand after juicing, or juice it if your machine handles seeds well. The result? A bold and tangy temptress of a drink.

Storage:

Pour into a sealed glass bottle and refrigerate for up to 3 days. The flavours deepen as they chill, so she only gets sassier with time.

To Serve:

Serve in a short cocktail glass or boba cup over ice. Add a lime wedge or passionfruit half on the rim. Warning: may cause sudden urges to sing to passing sailors.

*Tart, tangy, and totally irresistible like every good siren should be.

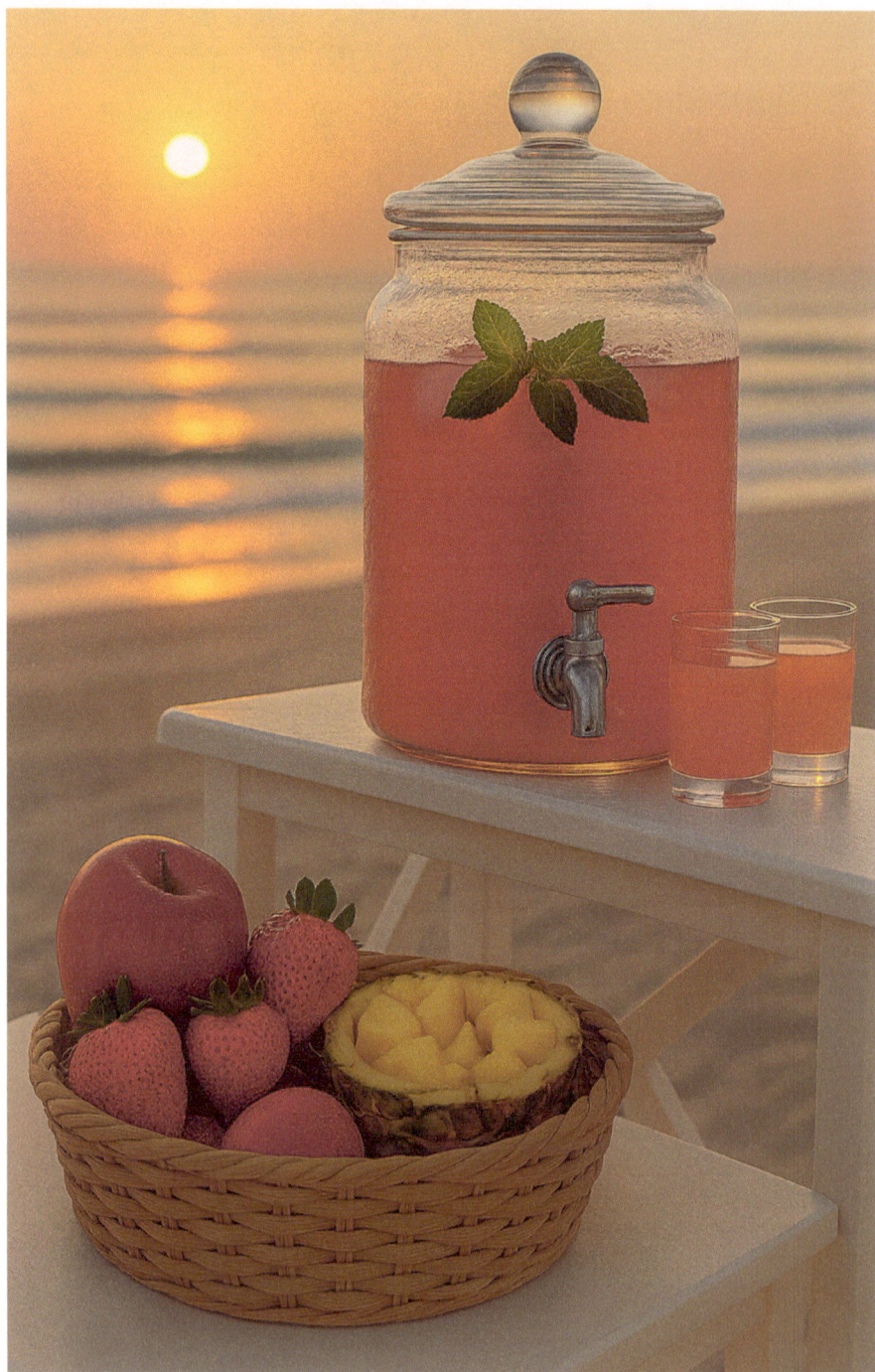

Sunset Kiss

Ingredients:

- 1 cup pineapple chunks
- 1 cup strawberries (hulled)
- 1 red apple (sweet variety)

Method:

Juice the apple and pineapple first for a tropical base, then follow with the strawberries for that sweet blush of colour. Use a cold press juicer to keep every sip smooth and golden.

Storage:

Pour into a chilled glass bottle and store in the fridge. This fruity fling stays fresh and flirty for 2 to 3 days.

To Serve:

Serve in a curvy glass or a mason jar with a heart-shaped straw and a strawberry slice on the rim. Best enjoyed at golden hour with someone (or something) you love.

*Sweet, juicy, and just a little bit cheeky like the perfect sunset kiss.

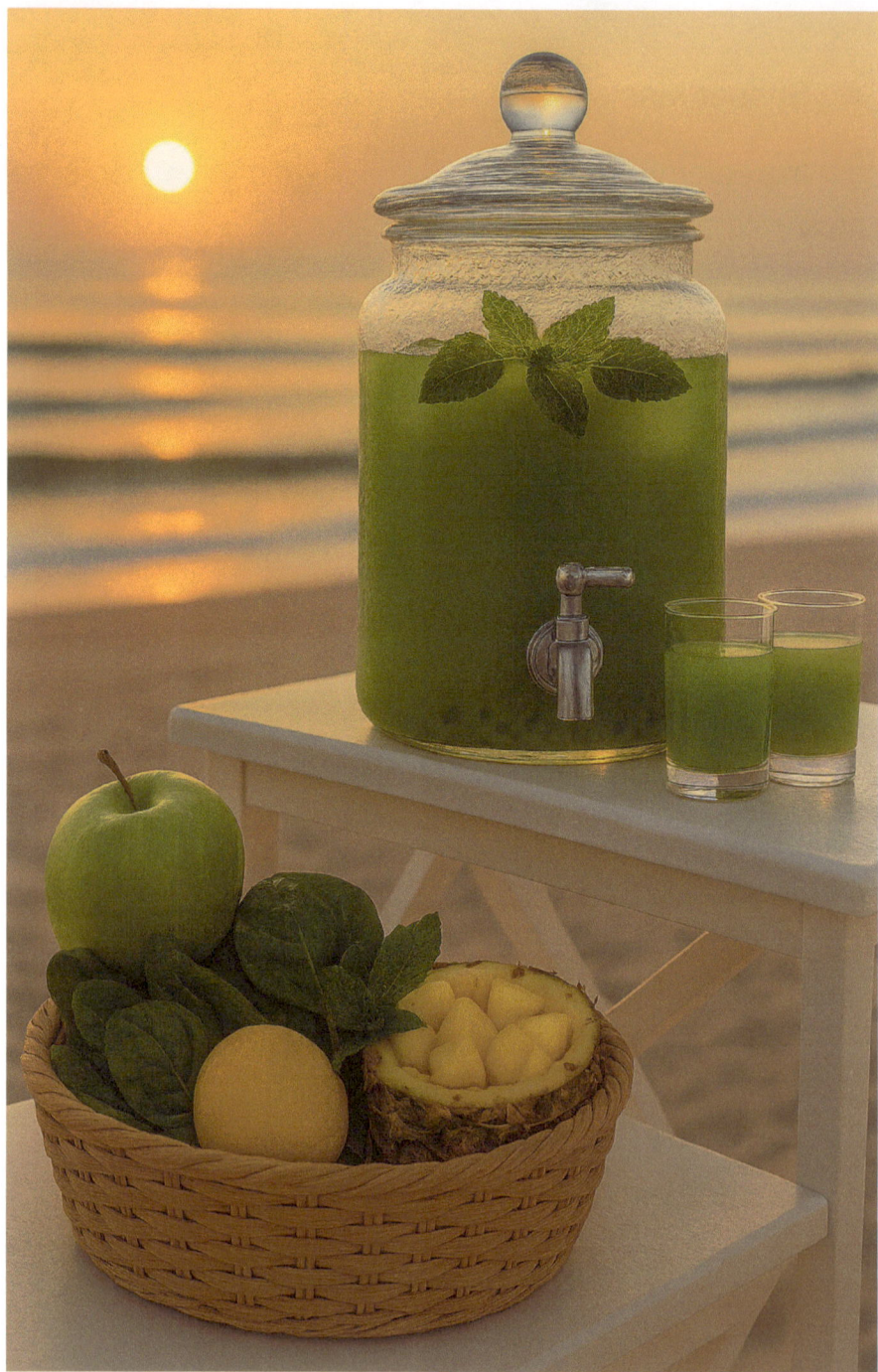

Wicked Wave

Ingredients:

- 1 green apple
- 1 handful of fresh mint leaves
- 1 handful of baby spinach
- 1/2 lemon (peeled, seeds removed)
- 1 cup pineapple chunks

Method:

Start by cold pressing the mint and spinach together to form the leafy foundation. Follow with the lemon, apple and finish strong with the juicy pineapple. This combo delivers a wave of zing and green goodness.

Storage:

Store in a sealed glass juice bottle in the fridge.
Wickedly fresh for up to 3 days but best enjoyed within 48 hours while the mint is still mischievous.

To Serve:

Serve in a highball glass with crushed ice and a mint sprig.
Optional: add a little umbrella, because why not?

* Bold, green, and just the right amount of wild ride the wave, babe.

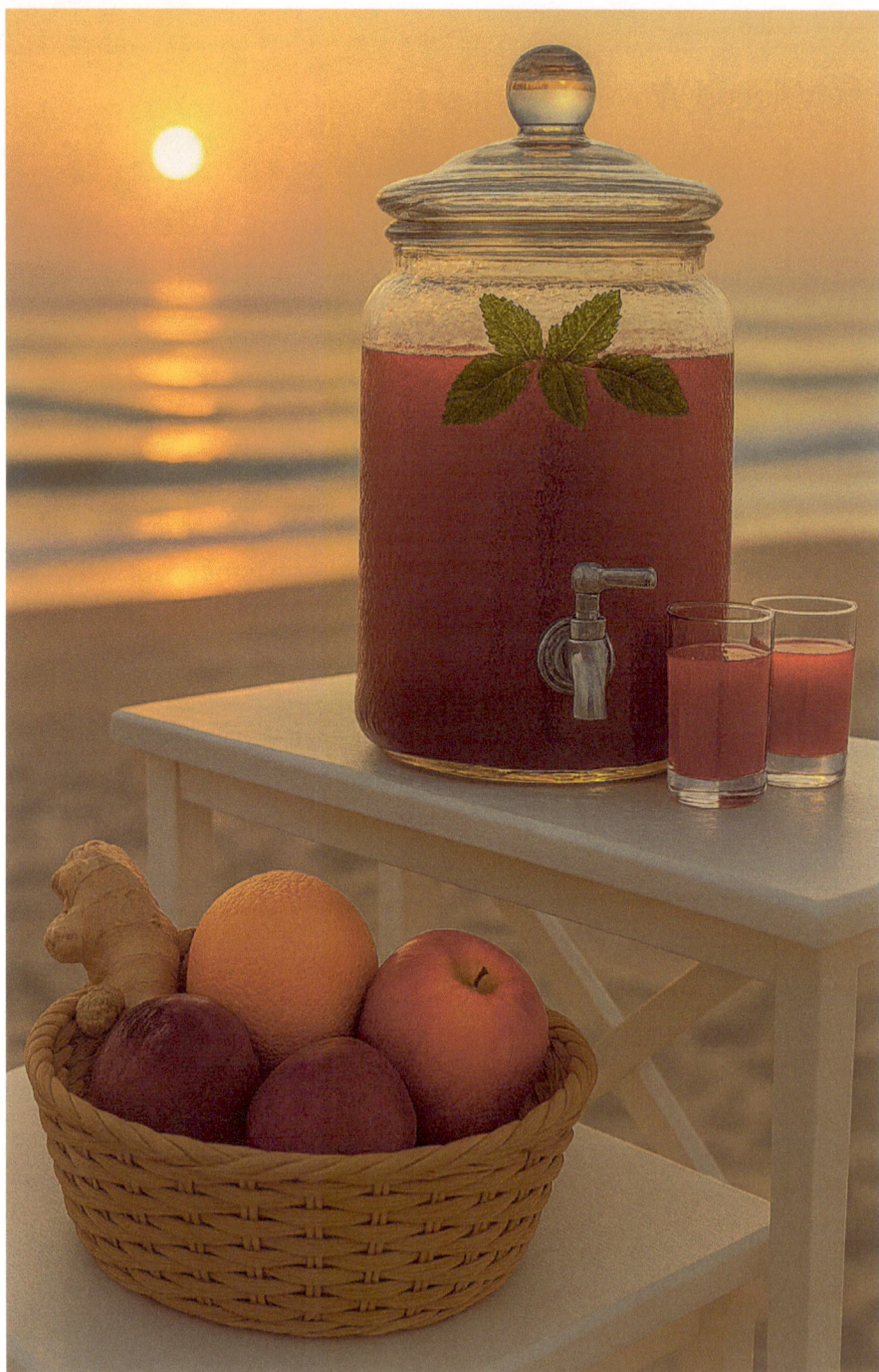

Crimson Current

Ingredients:

- 1 small knob of fresh ginger (about 1 inch, peeled)
- 1 small beetroot (peeled and quartered)
- 1 orange (peeled)
- 1 sweet red apple

Method:

1. Start by juicing the ginger and beetroot to build that rich, spicy base.
2. Then add the orange and apple to brighten the flavour with natural sweetness.
3. Use a cold press juicer to preserve the vibrant colour and full-bodied flavour.

Storage:

Store in a glass bottle with a secure lid. This juice holds its bold hue and flavour for up to 3 days in the fridge.

To Serve:

Serve chilled in a short glass or coupe over ice. Garnish with a twist of orange peel or a thin beetroot slice for that dramatic touch.

*Deep, bold, and unforgettable current worth getting swept up in.

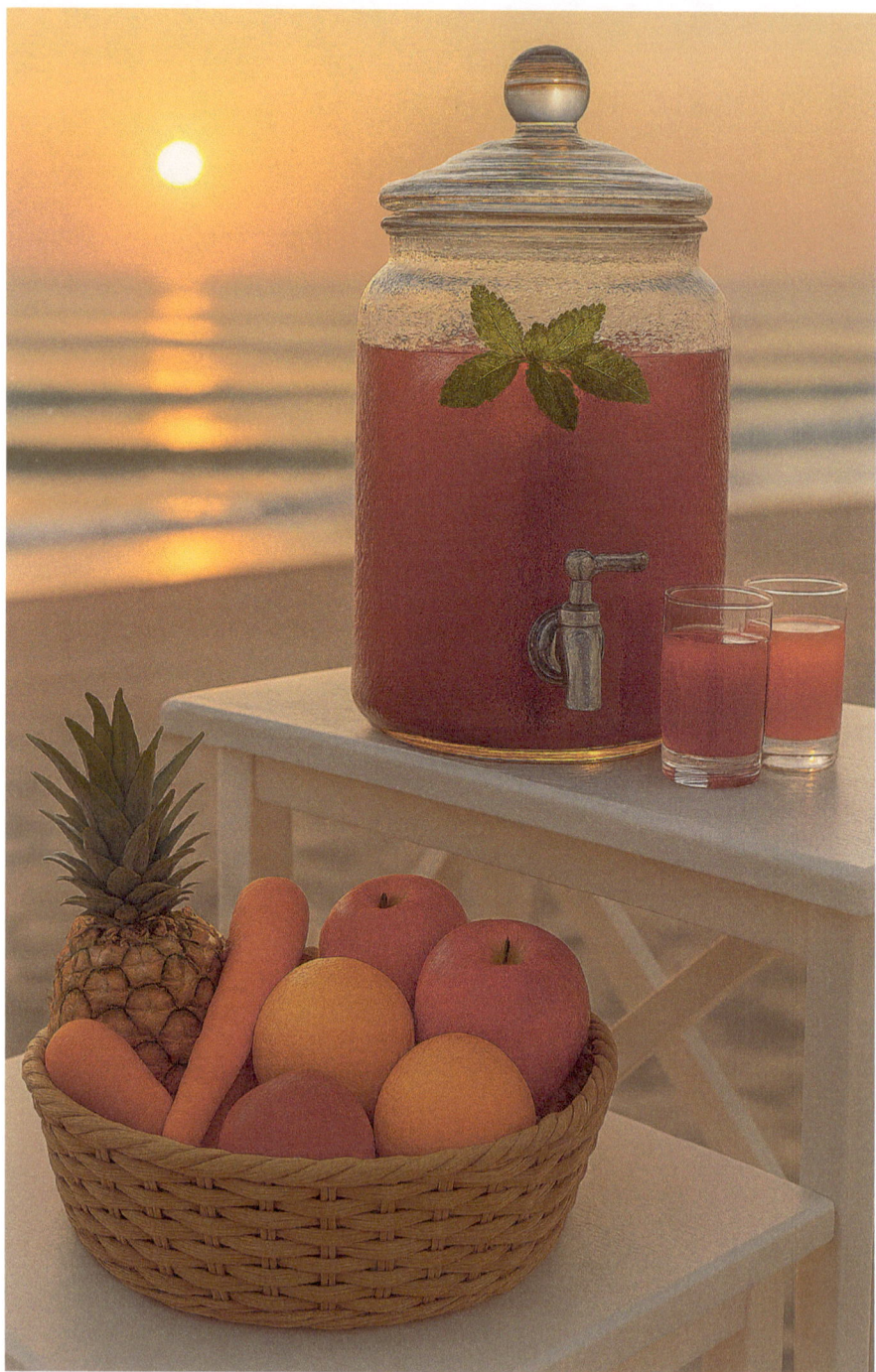

Lifeguard Elixir

Ingredients:

- 1 sweet red apple
- 1 small beetroot (peeled and quartered)
- 1 orange (peeled)
- 1 medium carrot (peeled)
- 1 small knob fresh ginger (about 1 inch, peeled)

Method:

1. Cold-press each ingredient starting with the beetroot and ginger, followed by carrot, orange, and apple.
2. This juice layers earthy depth with bright citrus and a hint of spicy warmth, just what your body ordered.

Storage:

Store in a 1L glass bottle in the fridge. It's best enjoyed within 2 to 3 days while it's still vibrant and full of rescue energy.

To Serve:

Serve over ice in a tall tumbler with a citrus wheel or carrot ribbon for flair. It's a lifeguard in liquid form.

Packed with colour, power, and a zesty punch, this is your wellness whistle in a cup.

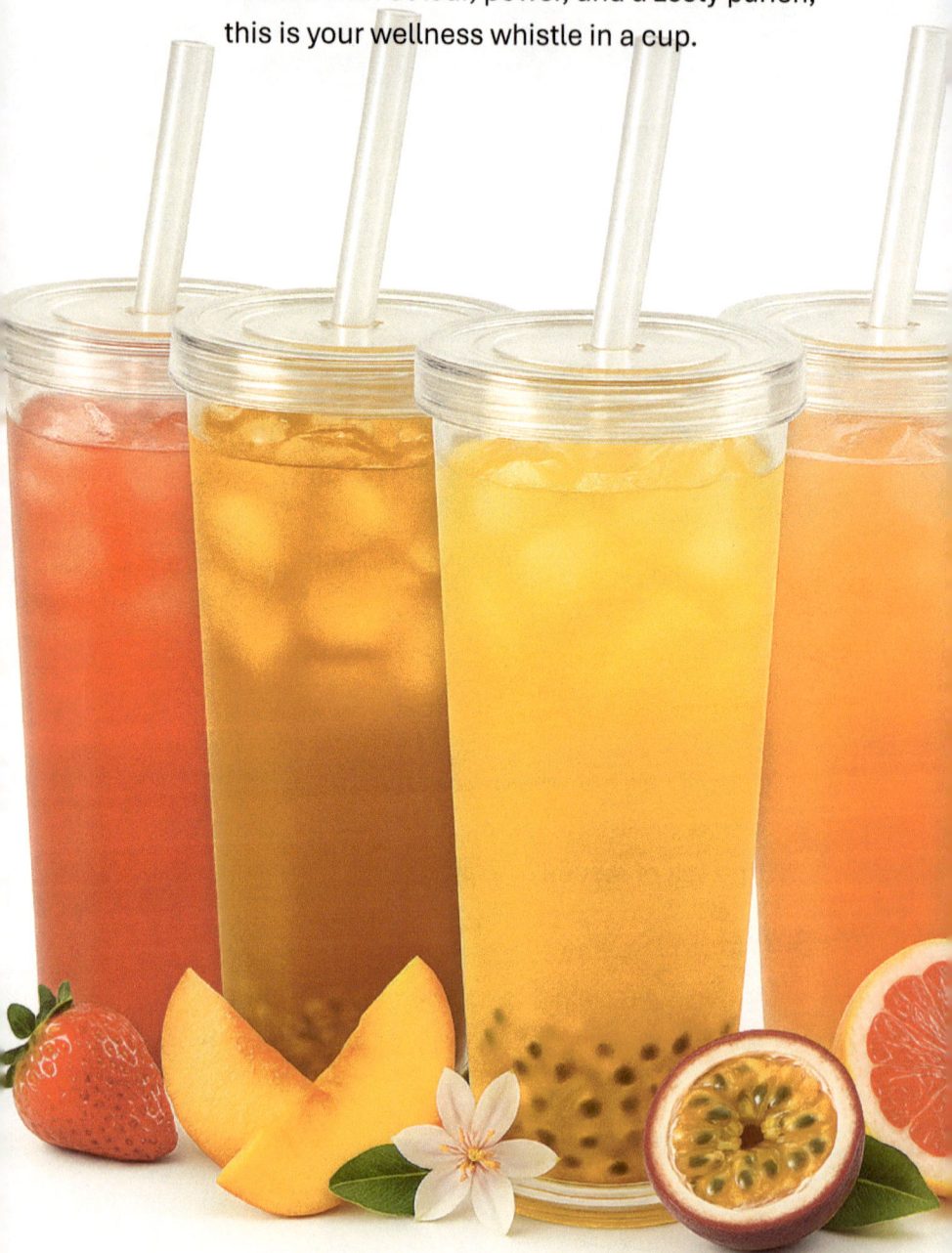

Boba Teas

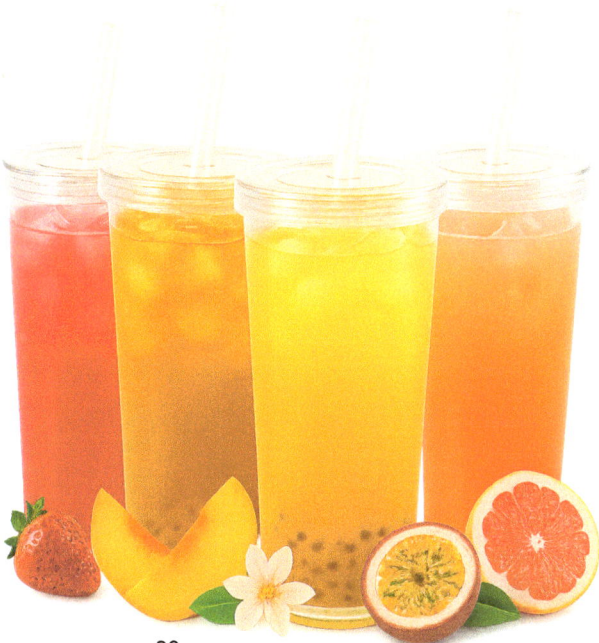

Glow Bar Boba Teas

Choose any flavour combination after the recipe card

*Juicy, bright refresher that's equal parts sweet and sassy. *

Ingredients:

- 1 cup organic caffeine-free green tea (brewed and chilled) or Oolong
- 2 tbsp of your favourite zero-sugar, gluten-free syrup
- ¼ cup fresh crushed fruits
- A generous handful of ice
- A scoop of your favourite boba pearls or jelly

Method:

Brew + Chill: Start by brewing your green tea and letting it cool completely. You want it crisp and cold, not lukewarm and moody. Fruit Fusion: In your serving cup, add the crushed fruit and syrup. Stir together to release that gorgeous blush. Add the Glow: Drop in your boba pearls or jelly, then fill the glass with ice.

Pour + Serve: Pour the chilled tea over the top and give it a gentle swirl. Sip in Style: Serve in a glass boba cup with a wide straw, bonus points if you're poolside in a sunhat.

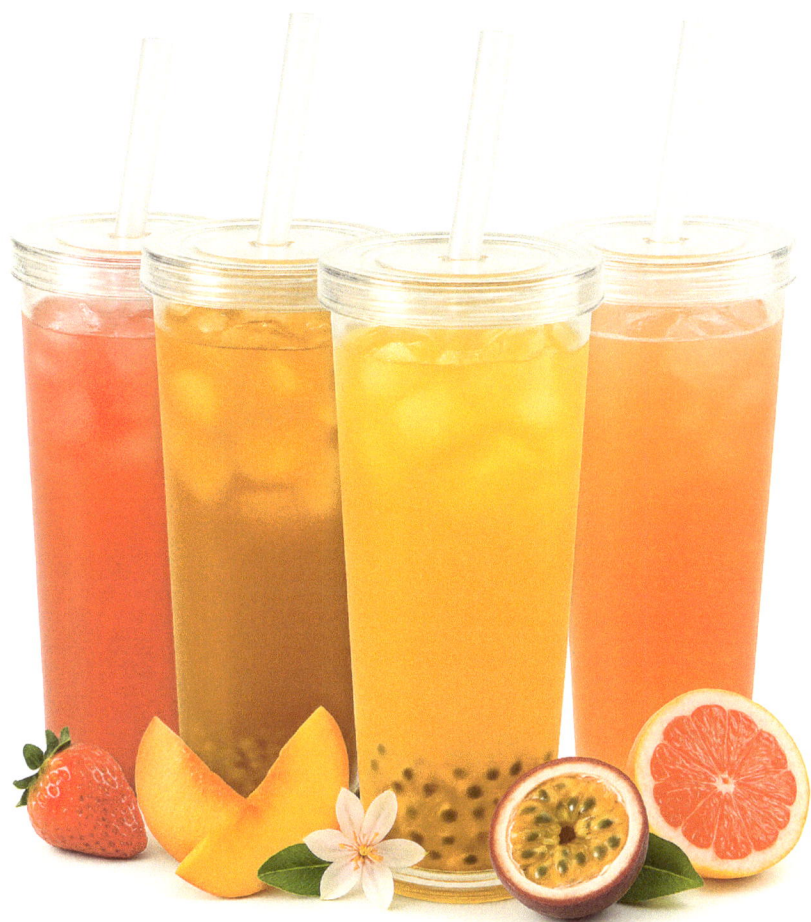

Double Strawberry Green

Ingredients:

- Organic caffeine-free green tea
- Your favourite zero-sugar, gluten-free strawberry syrup
- Crushed strawberries
- Ice
- Your favourite pearls or jelly

Method:

1. Brew your tea ahead and let it chill.
2. Add your fruit, syrup, and pearls.

To Serve:

Pour over ice and stir. Glow and go!

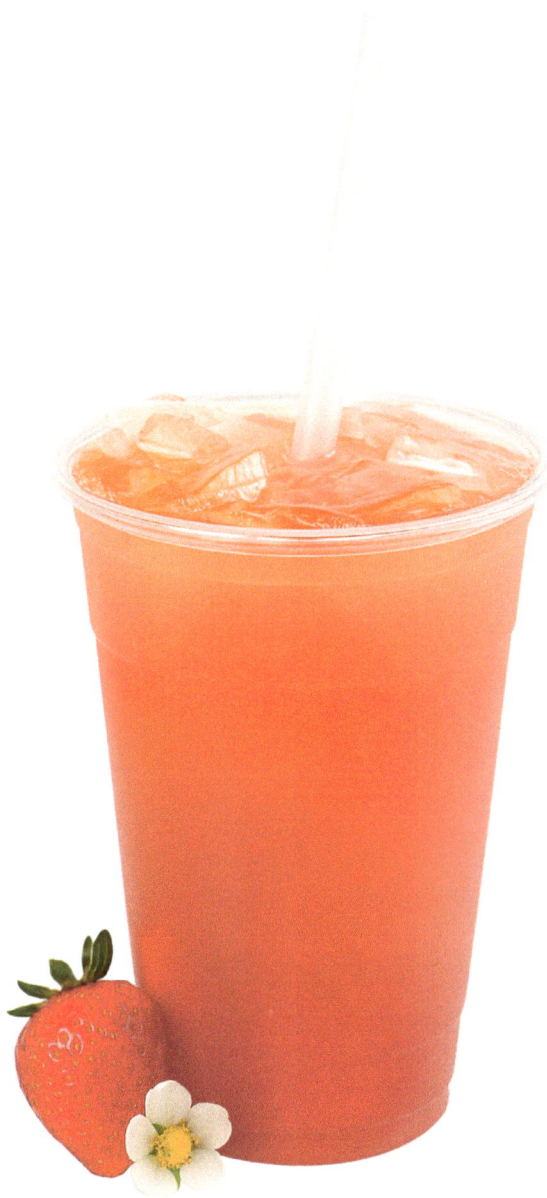

Peach Green Tea

Ingredients:

- Organic caffeine-free green tea
- Your favourite zero-sugar, gluten-free peach syrup
- Ice
- Your favourite pearls or jelly

Method:

1. Brew your tea ahead and let it chill.
2. Add your fruit, syrup, and pearls.

To Serve:

Pour over ice and stir. Glow and go!

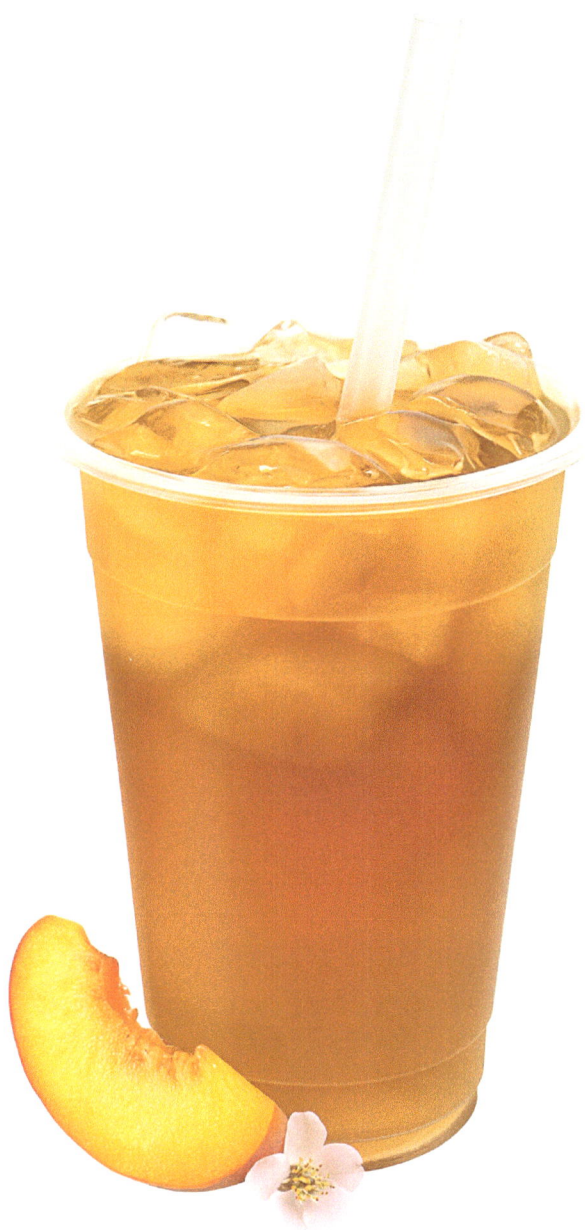

Grapefruit Green Tea

Ingredients:

- Organic caffeine-free green tea
- Your favourite zero-sugar, gluten-free grapefruit syrup
- Crushed grapefruit
- Ice
- Your favourite pearls or jelly

Method:

1. Brew your tea ahead and let it chill.
2. Add your fruit, syrup, and pearls.

To Serve:

Pour over ice and stir. Glow and go!

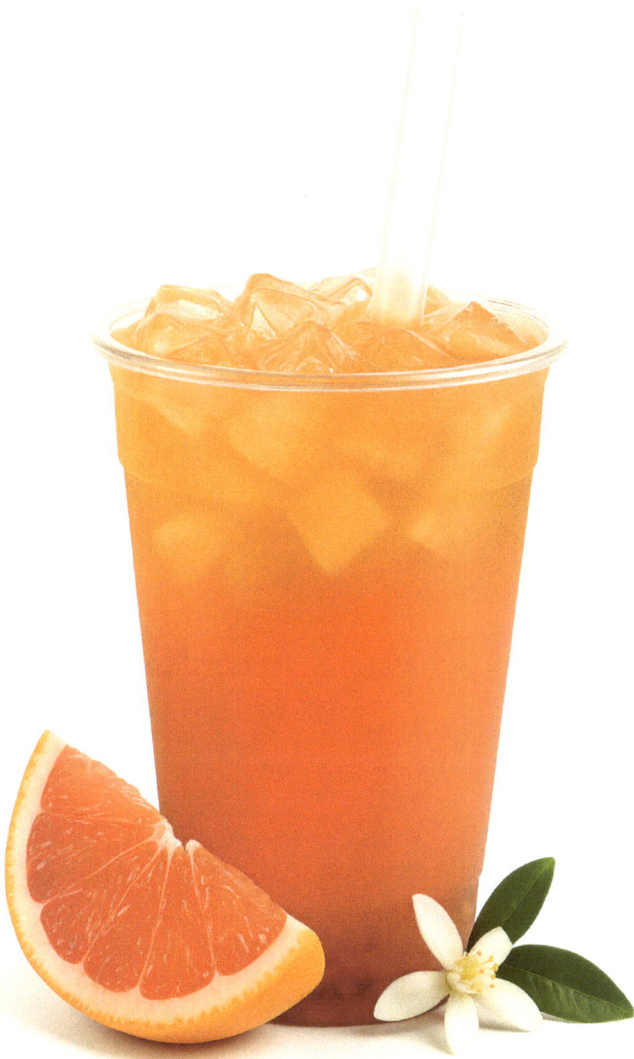

Passionfruit Green Tea

Ingredients:

- Organic caffeine-free oolong tea
- Your favourite zero-sugar, gluten-free passionfruit syrup
- Fresh Passion fruit
- Ice
- Your favourite pearls or jelly

Method:

Brew your tea ahead and let it chill. Add your fruit, syrup, and pearls.

To Serve:

Pour over ice and stir. Glow and go!

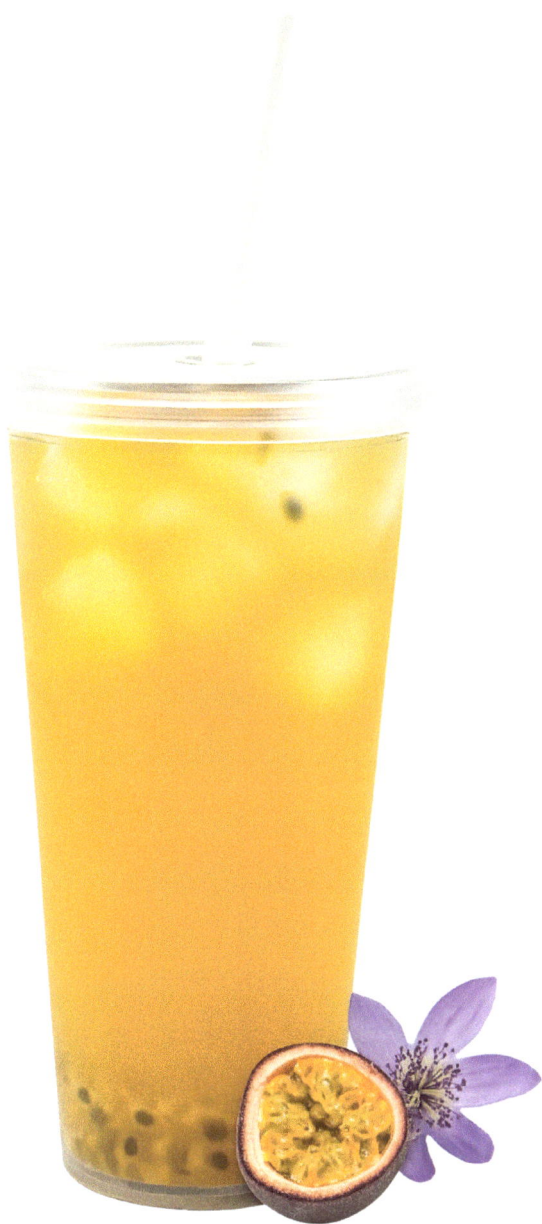

Lychee Oolong & Aloe

Ingredients:

- Organic caffeine-free oolong tea
- Your favourite zero-sugar, gluten-free lychee syrup
- Crushed lychee and aloe
- Ice
- Your favourite pearls or jelly

Method:

1. Brew your tea ahead and let it chill. Add your fruit, syrup, and pearls.

To Serve:

Pour over ice and stir. Glow and go!

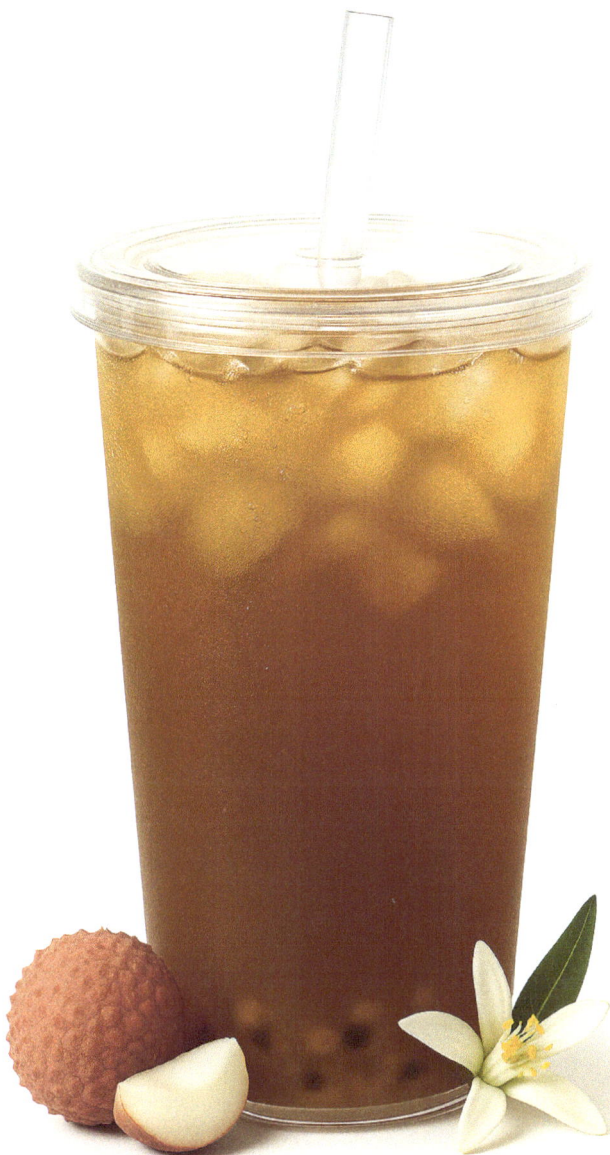

Mango Oolong

Ingredients:

- Organic caffeine-free oolong tea
- Your favourite zero-sugar, gluten-free mango syrup
- Ice
- Your favourite pearls or jelly

Method:

1. Brew your tea ahead and let it chill.
2. Add your fruit, syrup, and pearls.

To Serve:

Pour over ice and stir. Glow and go!

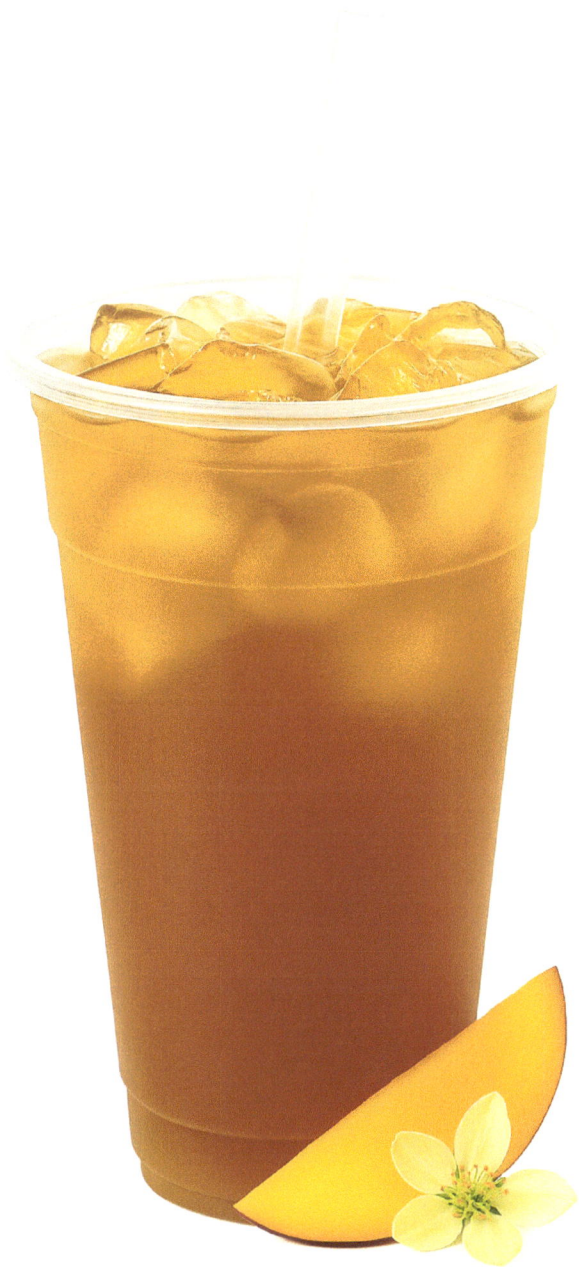

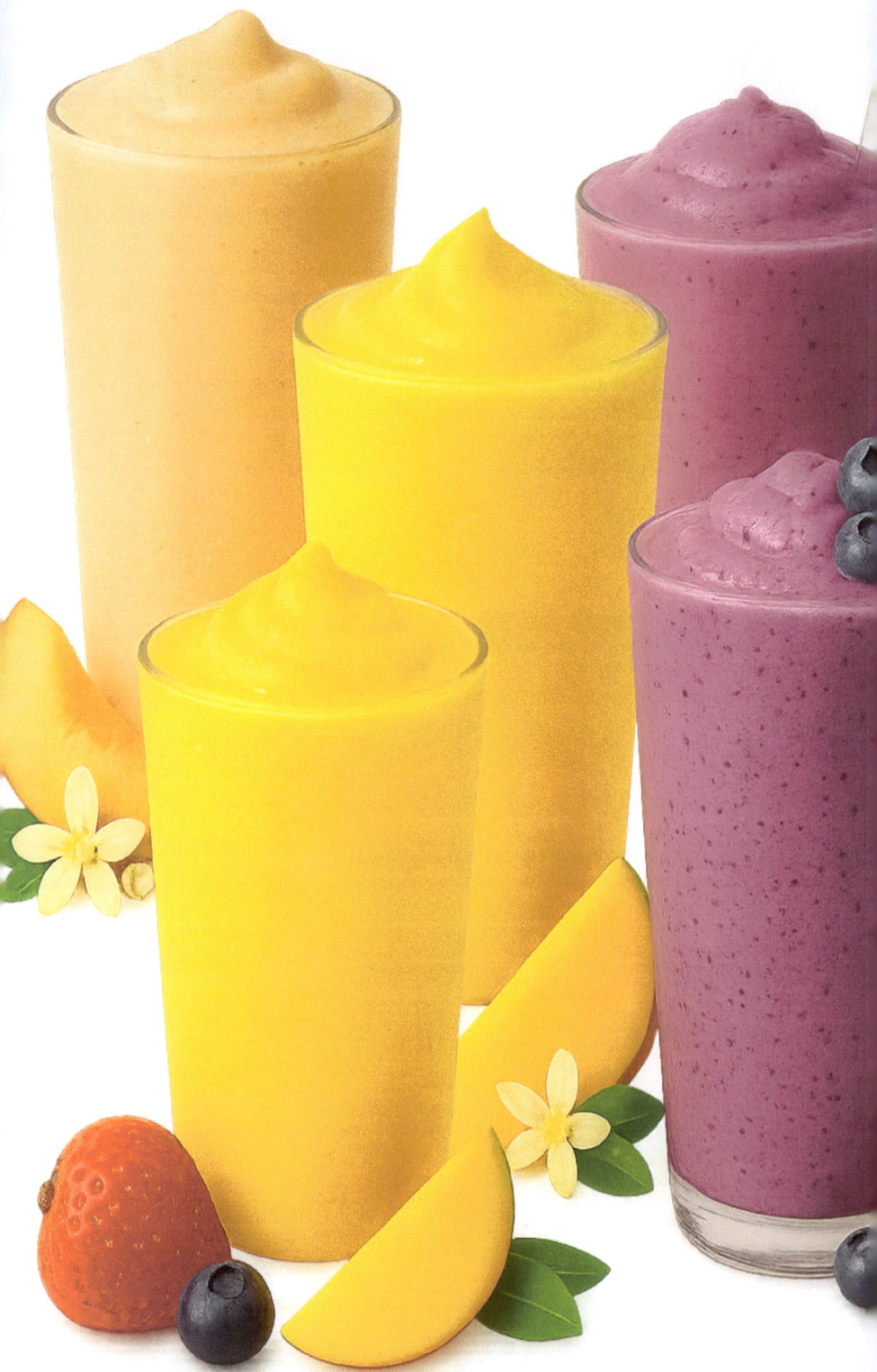

Smoothies

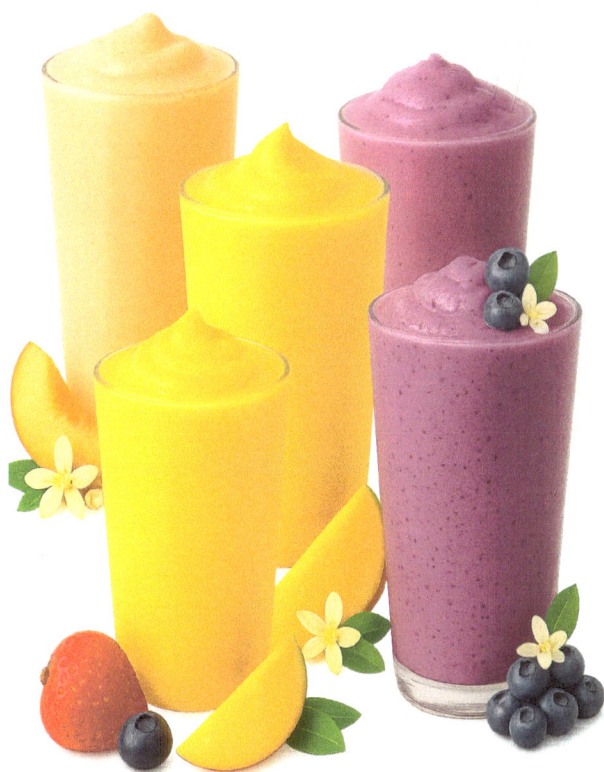

Peach Yoghurt Smoothie

Ingredients:

- 1/2 cup gluten-free coconut yogurt or Greek yogurt
- 1/2 cup almond milk or your favourite milk
- 1 cup fresh or frozen peaches
- 1 teaspoon Queen's vanilla paste

Method:

1. Add all ingredients to a blender and blend until smooth and creamy.
2. Add more milk if you prefer a thinner consistency or a handful of ice for a cooler, thicker smoothie.

To Serve:

Pour into a chilled glass or smoothie cup. Garnish with a peach slice or a sprinkle of granola for a summery touch.

Creamy, dreamy, and bursting with peachy goodness, your glow-up in a glass.

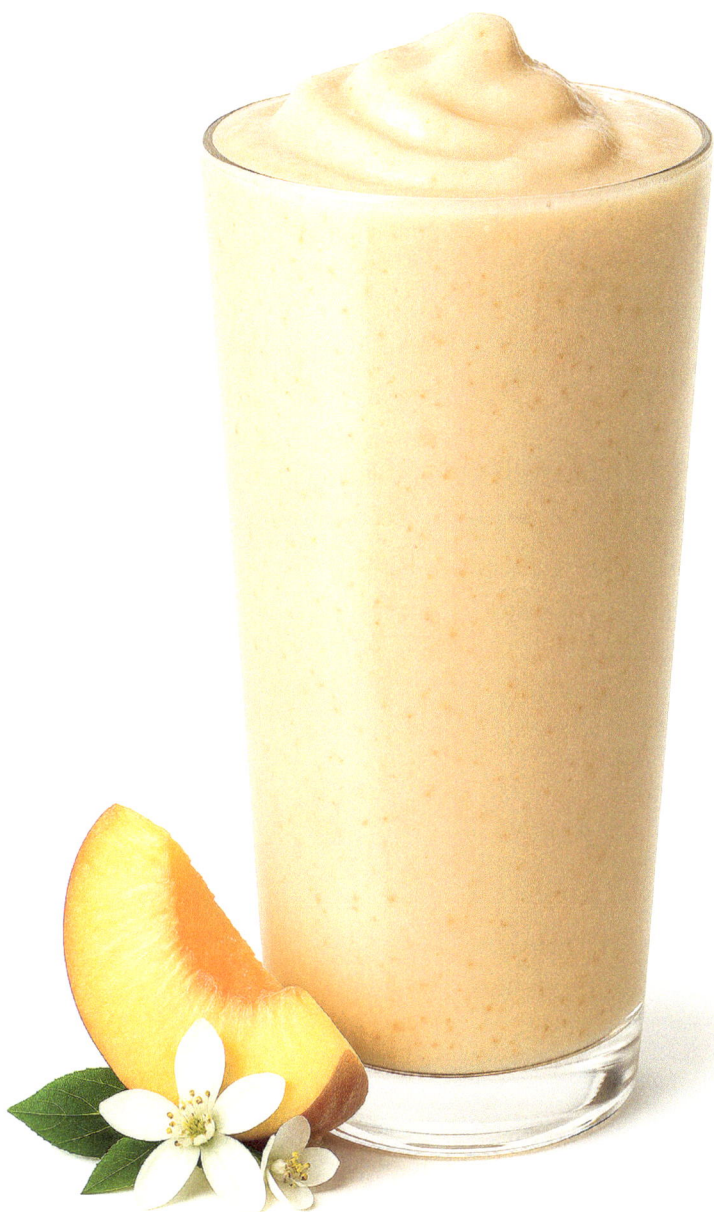

Mango Smoothie

Ingredients:

- 1/2 cup gluten-free coconut yogurt or Greek yogurt
- 1/2 cup almond milk or your favourite milk
- 1 cup fresh or frozen mango
- 1 teaspoon Queen's vanilla paste

Method:

1. Blend all ingredients in a high-speed blender until silky smooth.
2. Add more milk if you prefer a lighter consistency, or toss in a few ice cubes for that thick, frosty finish.

To Serve:

Serve chilled in your favourite tumbler or jar. Top with mango chunks or a mint leaf if you're feeling fancy.

Tropical, creamy, and sunshine in every sip, welcome to smoothie bliss.

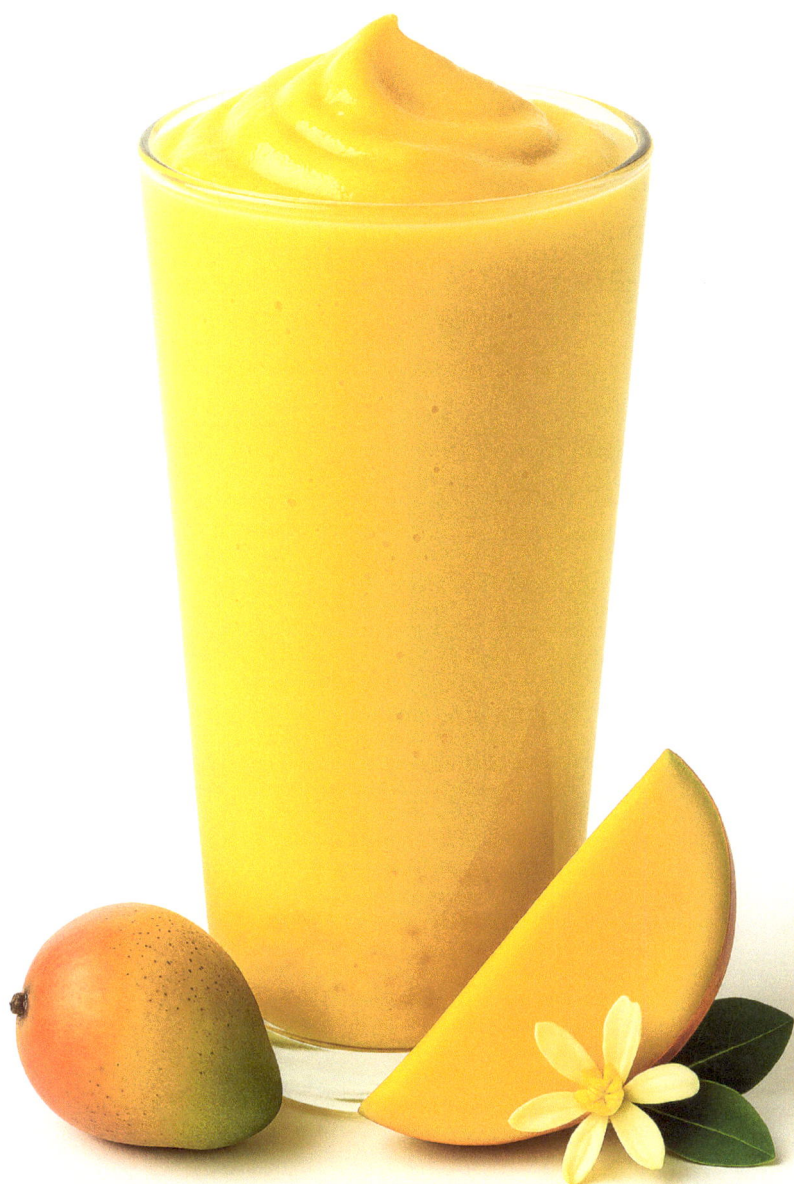

Mixed Berry Smoothie

Ingredients:

- 1/2 cup gluten-free coconut yogurt or Greek yogurt
- 1/2 cup almond milk or your favourite milk
- 1 cup fresh or frozen mixed berries
- 1 teaspoon Queen's vanilla paste

Method:

1. Place all ingredients into a blender and blend until smooth and vibrant.
2. Adjust the milk amount depending on how thick or sippable you want your smoothie.

To Serve:

Pour into a tall glass or smoothie cup. Top with a few whole berries or a sprinkle of chia seeds for extra flair.

Berry bold, beautifully balanced, and totally delicious, a smoothie that does it all.

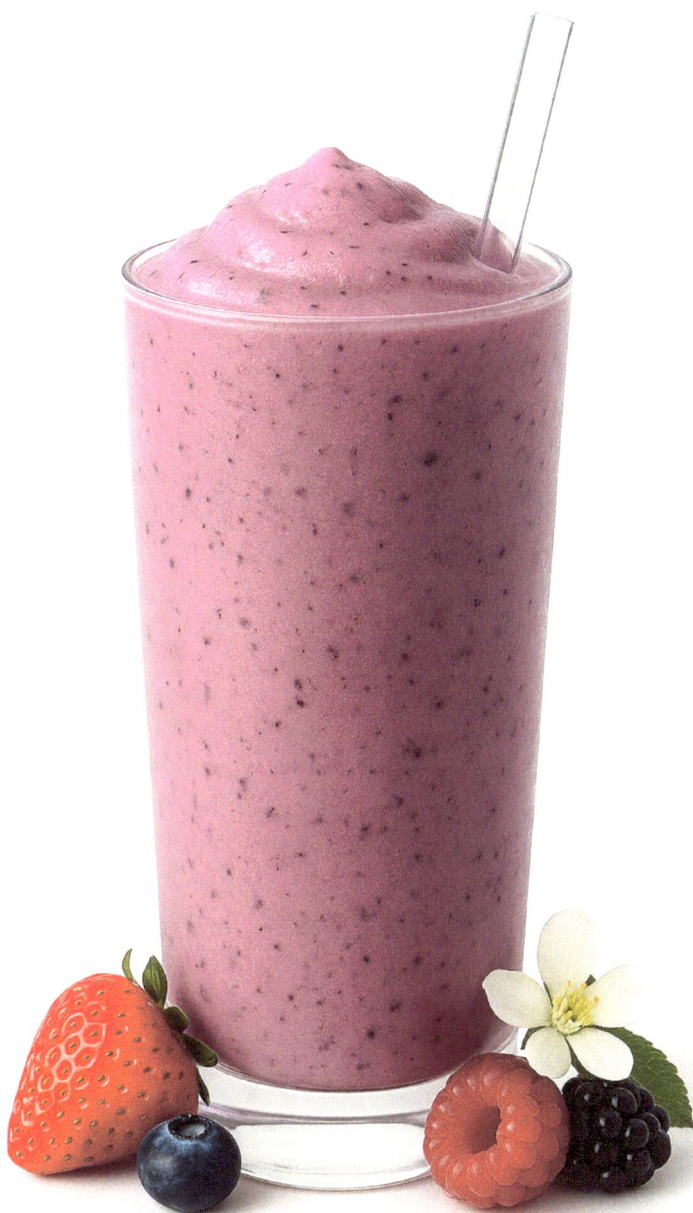

Blueberry Smoothie

Ingredients:

- 1/2 cup gluten-free coconut yogurt or Greek yogurt
- 1/2 cup almond milk or your favourite milk
- 1 cup fresh or frozen blueberries
- 1 teaspoon Queen's vanilla paste

Method:

1. Add all ingredients into your blender and blend until beautifully purple and creamy.
2. Add extra milk if needed to reach your perfect sipping consistency.

To Serve:

Serve in a chilled glass or smoothie jar. Top with a few blueberries or edible flowers for a luxe breakfast moment.

Silky, fruity, and full of brain-boosting glow, this is your blue-hued power potion.

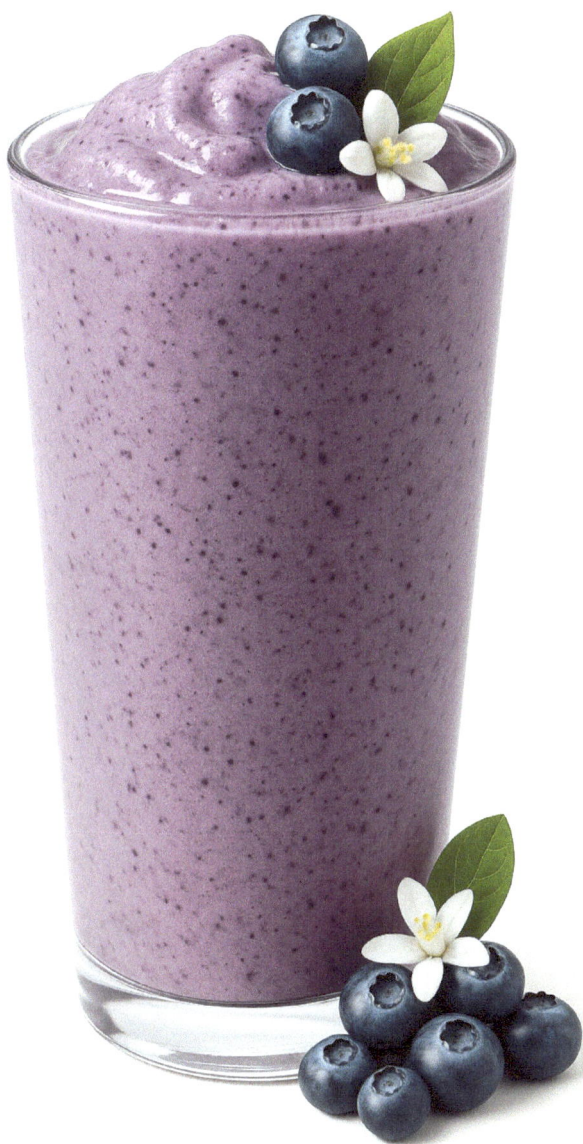

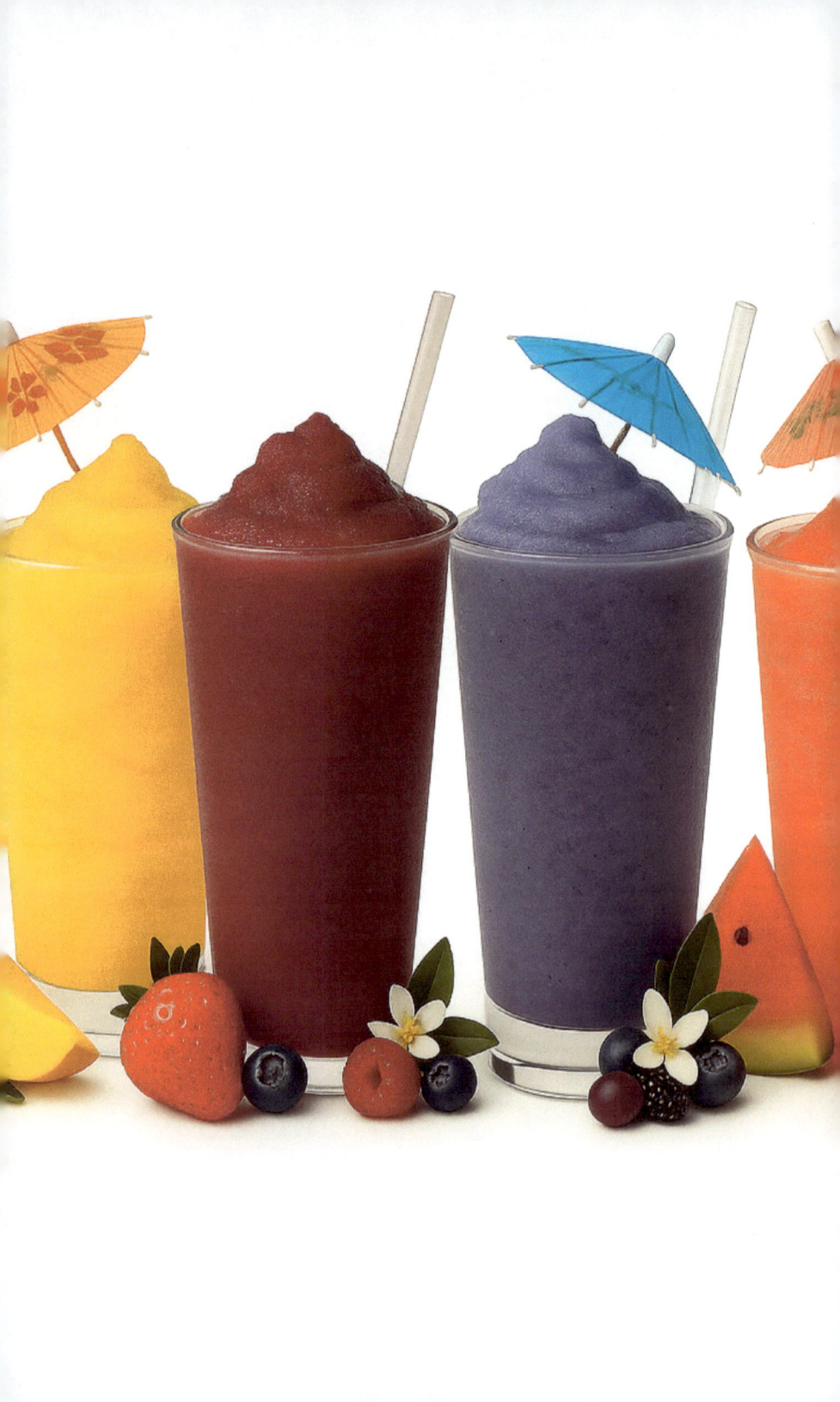

Frappes

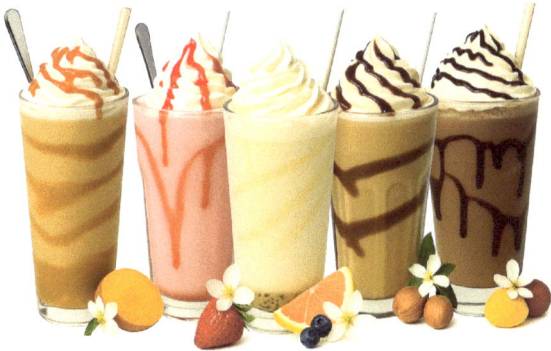

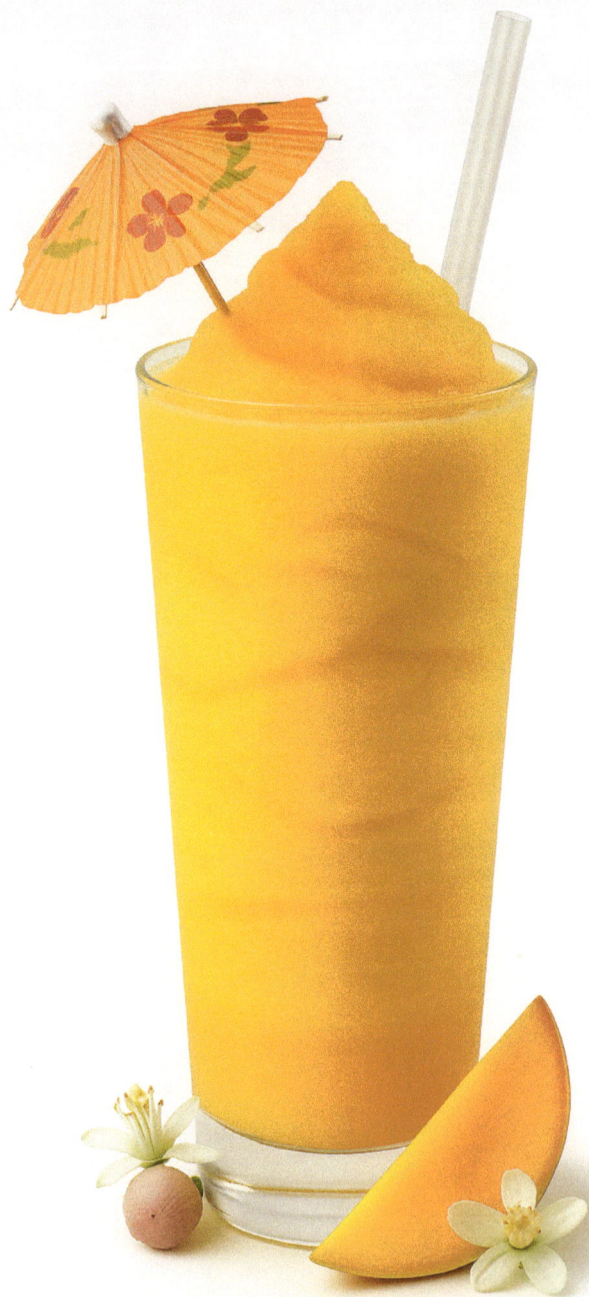

Mango Frappe

Ingredients:

- 1 cup ice
- 1 cup mango (50/50 mix of fresh or tinned and frozen mango)
- A few fresh spearmint leaves

Method:

1. Add the mango and ice to a blender and blend until icy and slushy.
2. Add the spearmint at the end and pulse gently to distribute the flavour without turning the drink green.

To Serve:

Pour into a chilled glass and garnish with a fresh spearmint sprig or a mango slice. Perfect for tropical daydreams.

Cool, zesty, and full of sunshine, your summer slushie fantasy awaits.

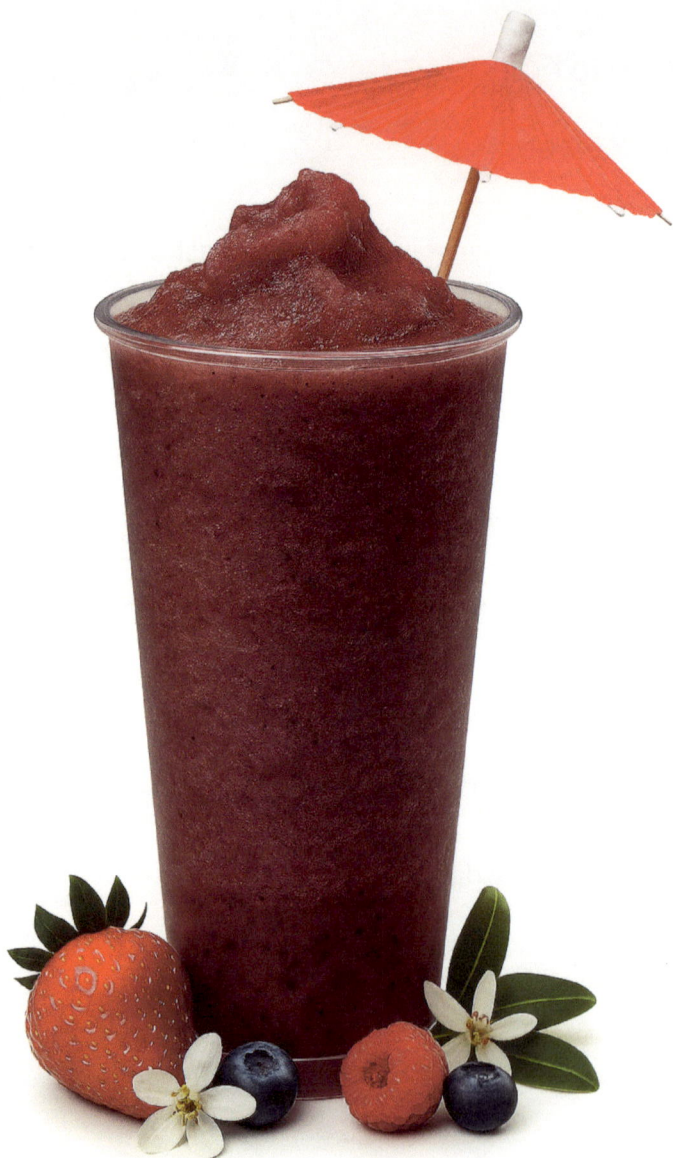

Mixed Berry Frappe

Ingredients:

- 1 cup ice
- 1 cup mixed berries (50/50 mix of fresh or tinned and frozen berries)
- A few fresh spearmint leaves

Method:

1. Add berries and ice to a blender and blend until thick and icy.
2. Drop in the spearmint and pulse briefly to keep it fresh and fragrant without overpowering the berries.

To Serve:

Serve in a frosty glass with a handful of whole berries on top and a sprig of spearmint. Sip slowly and pretend you're at a mountain spa with berry-stained lips.

Berry chilly, super pretty, and dangerously refreshing.

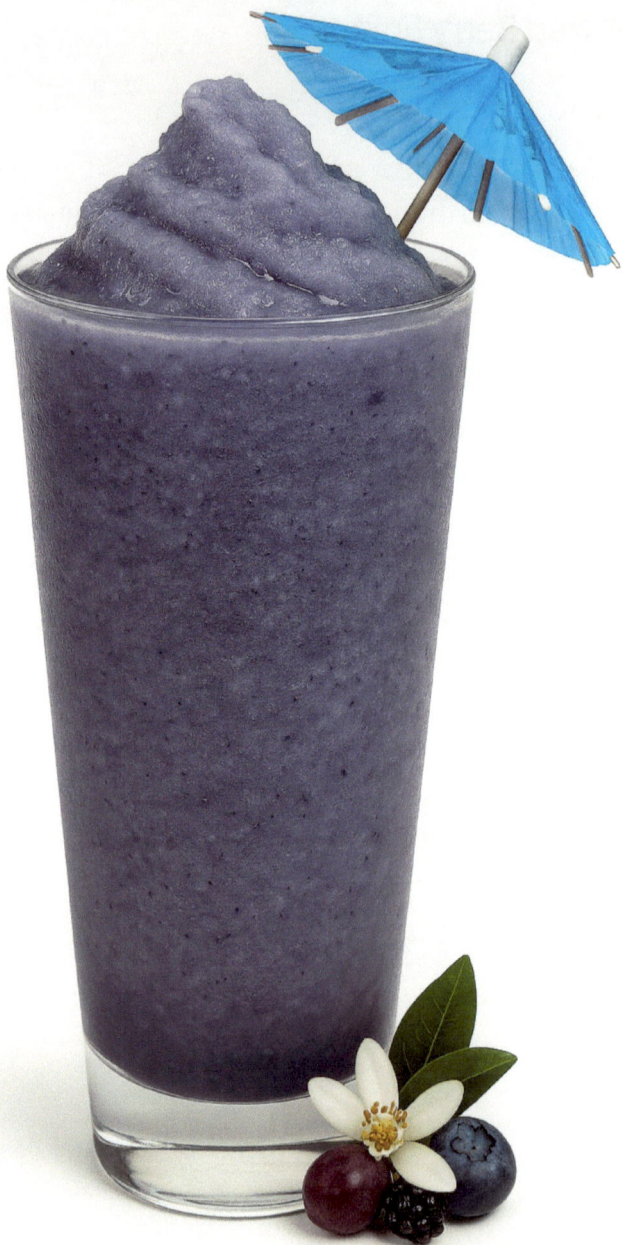

Blueberry Frappe

Ingredients:

- 1 cup ice
- 1 cup blueberries (50/50 mix of fresh or tinned and frozen berries)
- A few fresh spearmint leaves
- 1 tablespoon of your favourite zero-sugar, gluten-free vanilla syrup

Method:

1. Add blueberries and ice to your blender and blend until thick and icy.
2. Add the vanilla syrup and spearmint, then pulse once or twice to infuse without overpowering the berry goodness.

To Serve:

Serve in a chilled glass topped with a few blueberries and a tiny sprig of spearmint. Feels like a snowflake kissed by a blueberry.

Frosty, fragrant, and sweetened just right, your cool-girl crush in a glass.

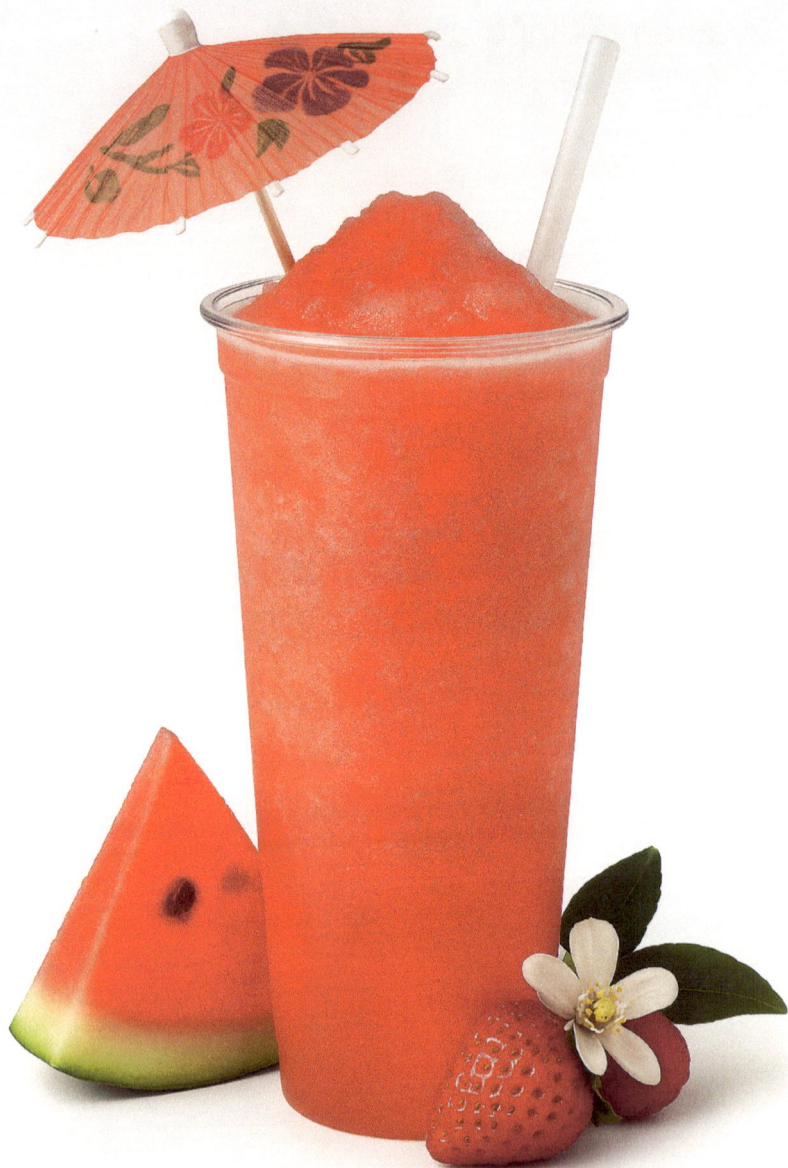

Watermelon Frappe

Ingredients:

- 1 cup ice
- 1 cup watermelon (50/50 mix of fresh or tinned and frozen)
- A few fresh spearmint leaves
- 1 tablespoon of your favourite zero-sugar, gluten-free watermelon syrup

Method:

1. Add watermelon and ice to the blender and blend until perfectly slushy.
2. Drizzle in your syrup and toss in the spearmint last.
3. Pulse once or twice to keep that crisp, refreshing flavour.

To Serve:

Pour into a chilled glass and top with a watermelon wedge and mint sprig. Extra cute with a paper umbrella and a poolside view.

Sweet, splashy, and cool as a beach breeze, the glow-up your summer deserves.

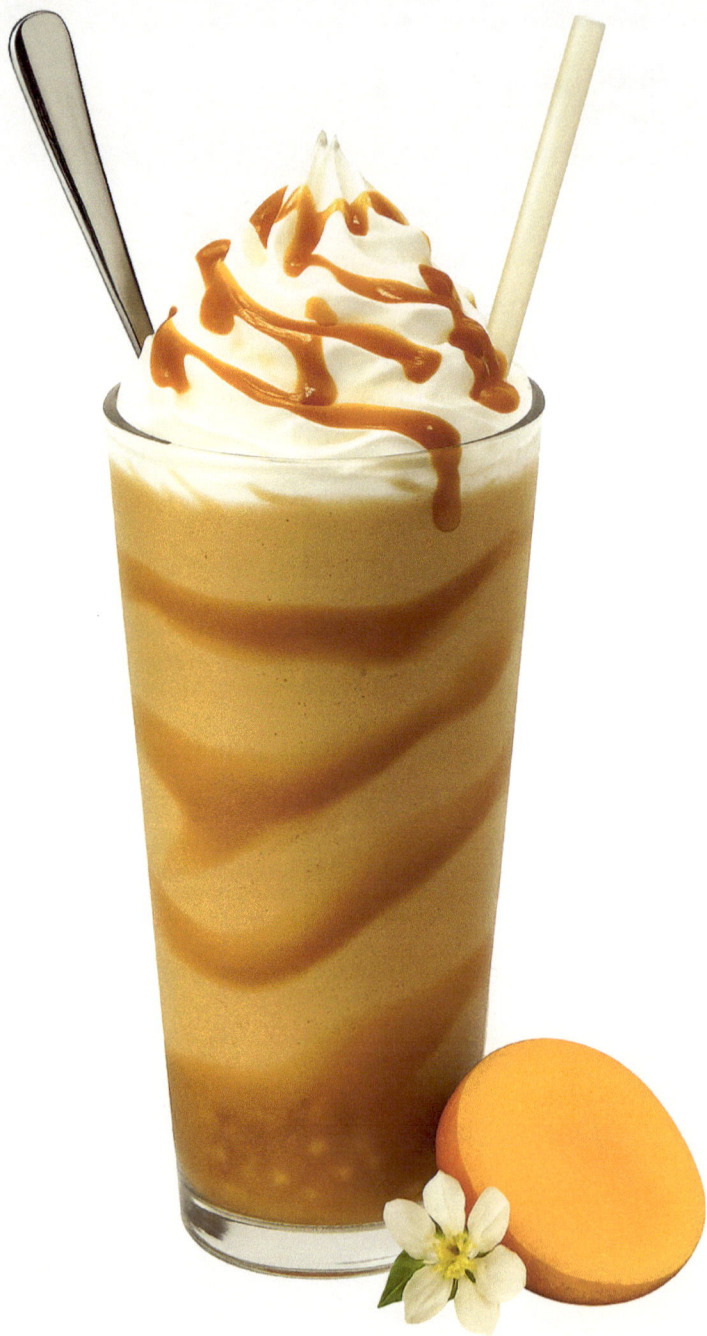

Caramel Frappe Milk

Ingredients:

- 1 tablespoon of your favourite zero-sugar, gluten-free caramel syrup
- 1 cup almond milk or your favourite milk
- 1 cup ice
- 1 drizzle of sugar-free salted caramel ice cream topping

Method:

1. Blend the caramel syrup, milk, and ice together until smooth and frothy.
2. Adjust the sweetness to taste by adding a touch more syrup if desired.

To Serve:

Pour into a tall glass or insulated tumbler. Drizzle the sugar-free salted caramel topping on top and give it a gentle swirl. Optional: top with whipped cream for a little extra indulgence.

Rich, cool, and silky smooth like a dessert that also hydrates.

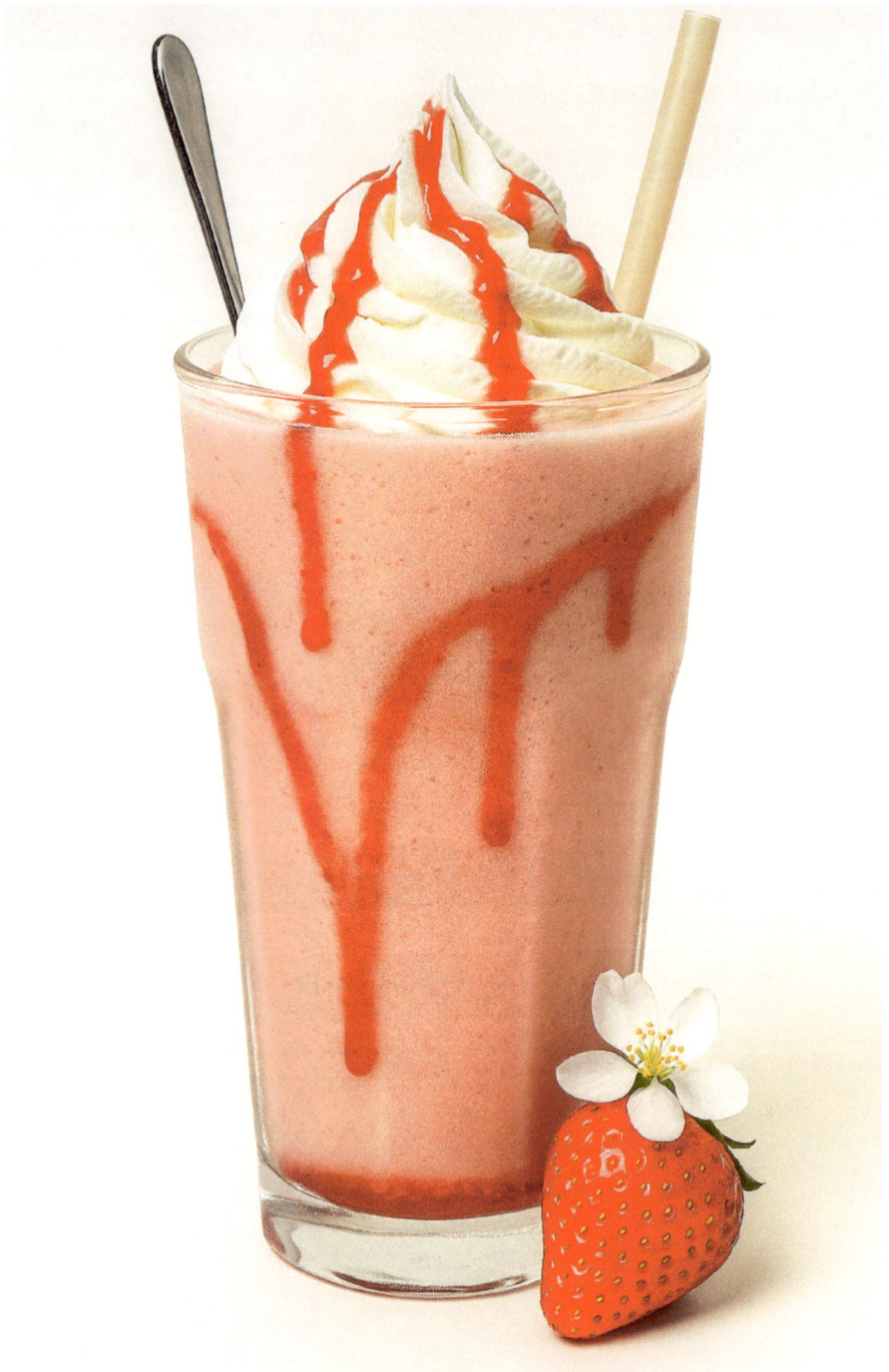

Strawberry Frappe Milk

Ingredients:

- 1 tablespoon of your favourite zero-sugar, gluten-free strawberry syrup
- 1 cup almond milk or your favourite milk
- 1 cup ice
- 1 drizzle of sugar-free, gluten-free strawberry ice cream topping

Method:

1. Blend the strawberry syrup, milk, and ice until smooth and frothy.
2. Add more syrup if you want it extra berry sweet.

To Serve:

Pour into a clear glass or travel cup. Drizzle the strawberry topping over the top and give it a little swirl. Perfect for pink-loving glow-getters.

Berry bright, ice-cold, and fabulously pink, this one's your sweet spa-day-in-a-glass.

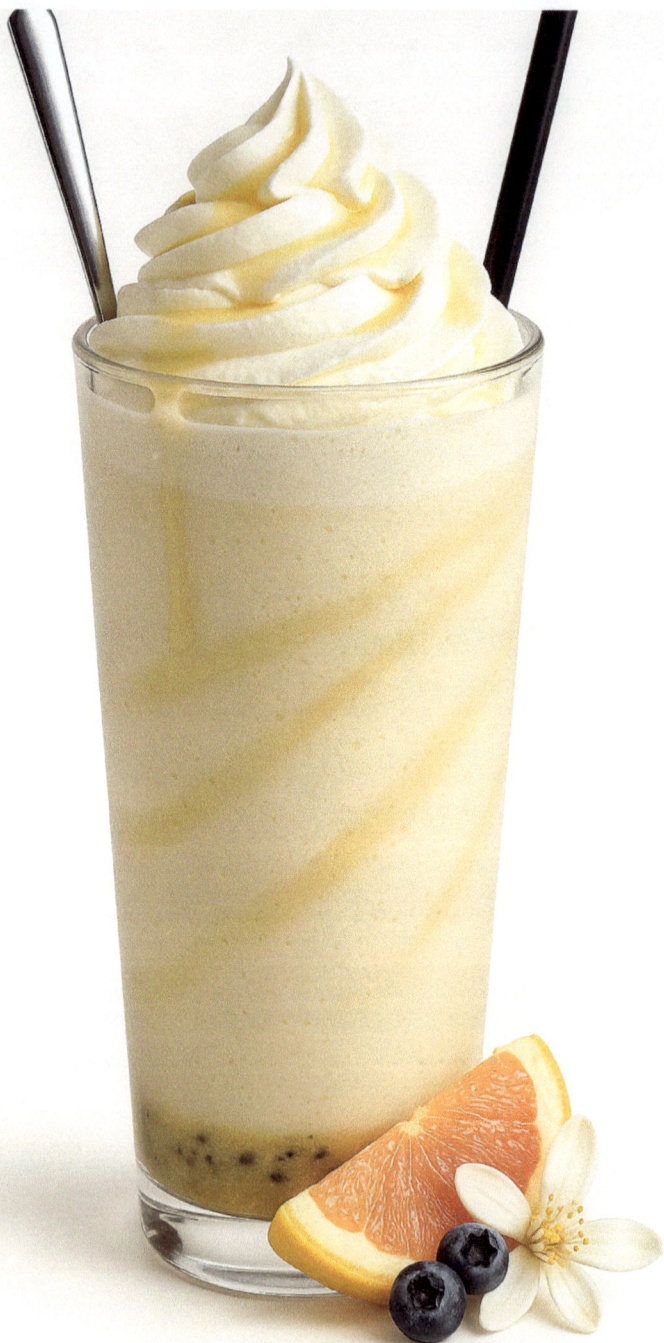

Vanilla Frappe Milk

Ingredients:

- 1 tablespoon of your favourite zero-sugar, gluten-free vanilla syrup
- 1 cup almond milk or your favourite milk
- 1 cup ice
- 1 drizzle of sugar-free, gluten-free vanilla-flavoured ice cream topping

Method:

1. Blend the vanilla syrup, milk, and ice until creamy and cloudlike.
2. Add extra ice for a thicker texture or more syrup if you like it sweeter.

To Serve:

Serve in a chilled glass or take-away style cup. Drizzle the vanilla topping over the surface for that dreamy dessert finish.

Light, luxe, and oh-so-smooth, this one's pure glow bar bliss in a glass.

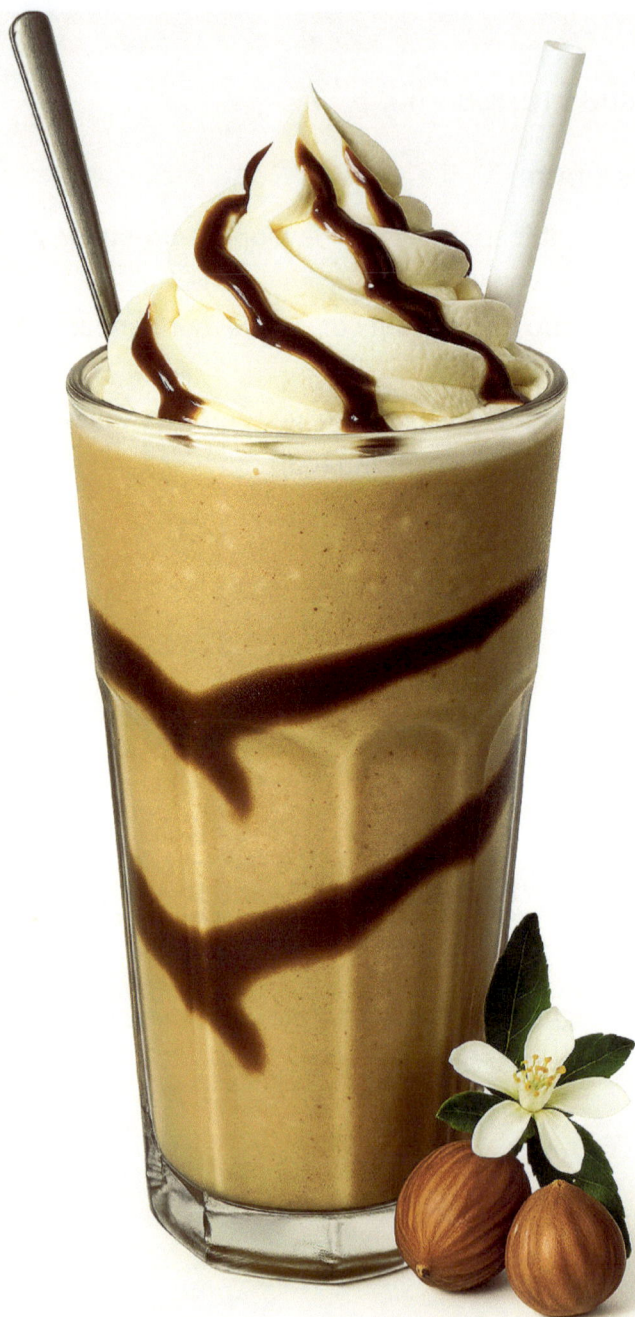

Hazelnut Frappe Milk

Ingredients:

- 1 tablespoon of your favourite zero-sugar, gluten-free hazelnut syrup
- 1 cup almond milk or your favourite milk
- 1 cup ice
- 1 heaped teaspoon of your favourite chocolate spread

Method:

1. Blend the hazelnut syrup, milk, chocolate spread, and ice until smooth and frothy.
2. Adjust sweetness and thickness to your liking by adding more syrup or ice.

To Serve:

Serve in a cozy mug or tall glass. Optional: drizzle extra chocolate spread on top or rim the glass for a glow-up-worthy indulgence.

Nutty, chocolatey, and decadent like a hug from your inner barista.

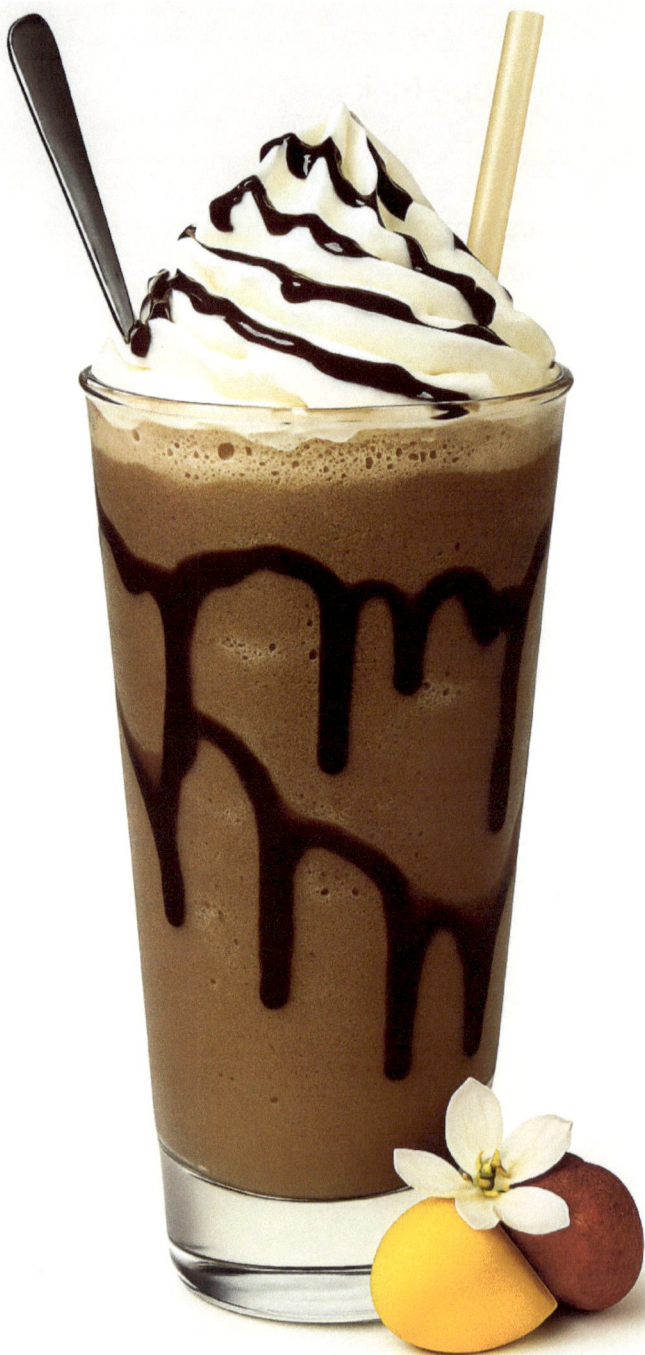

Mocha Frappe Milk

Ingredients:

- 1 tablespoon of your favourite zero-sugar, gluten-free hazelnut syrup
- 1 teaspoon caffeine-free instant coffee (or your favourite brewed coffee, cooled)
- 1 cup almond milk or your favourite milk
- 1 cup ice
- 1 heaped teaspoon of your favourite chocolate spread

Method:

1. Blend coffee, hazelnut syrup, milk, chocolate spread, and ice until cold and creamy.
2. Adjust intensity with more coffee or syrup to taste.

To Serve:

Serve in a tall glass or insulated tumbler. Garnish with a swirl of chocolate spread or a dusting of cocoa for that coffeehouse charm.

Cool, bold, and buzz-worthy, this mocha moment is pure glow bar energy.

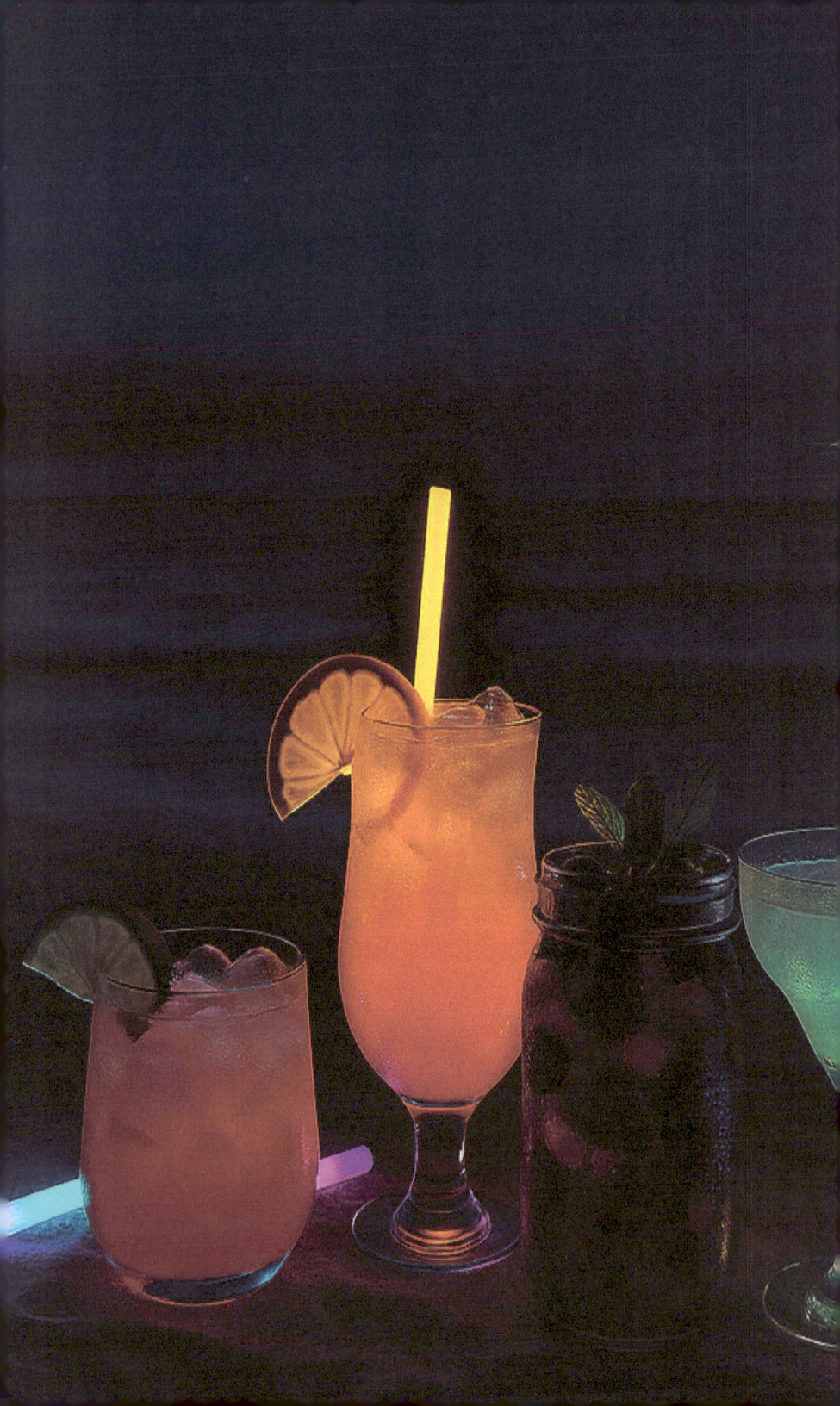

Glow Bar Cocktails

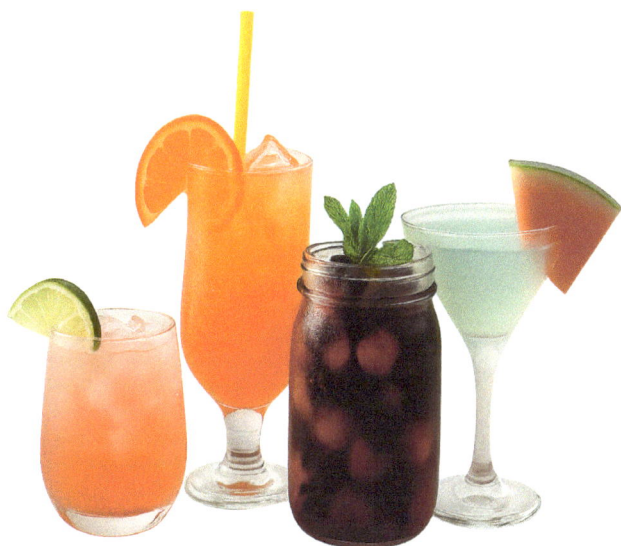

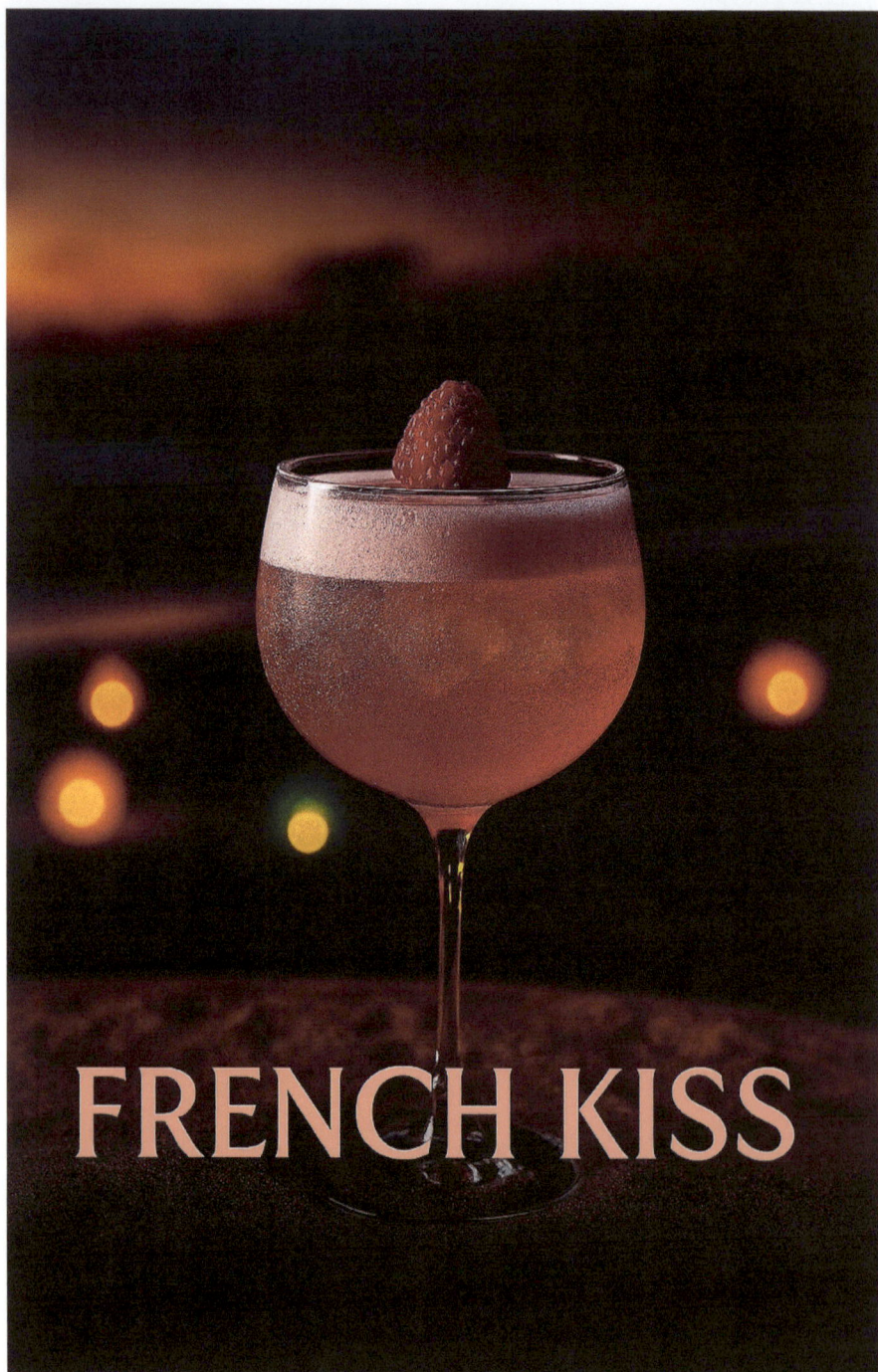

FRENCH KISS

French Kiss

A fizzy flirtation with lemon, berries, and just enough sparkle to make anyone blush.

Ingredients:

- Vodka
- Fresh lemon juice
- Simple syrup
- Chambord (or any raspberry liqueur)
- Prosecco
- Fresh raspberries (for garnish)
- Ice

Method:

1. Fill your cocktail shaker with ice, vodka, lemon juice, and simple syrup.
2. Shake it like you mean it passionately, but with grace.
3. Strain into a tall glass or champagne flute. Add a splash of Chambord, then top with prosecco.

To Serve:

Drop in a few fresh raspberries and let the romance begin.

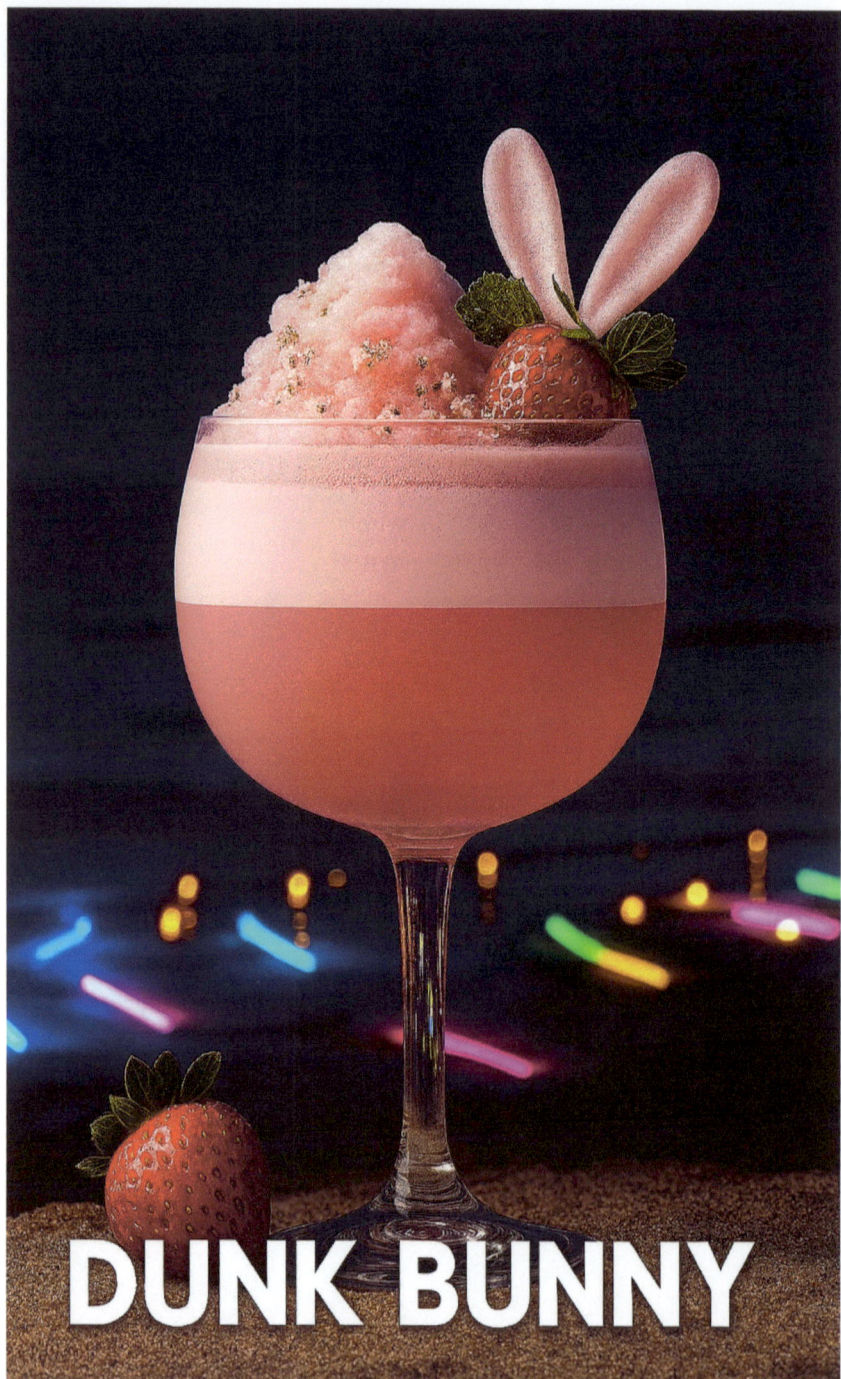

DUNK BUNNY

Dunk Bunny Cocktail

Ingredients:

- 2 oz coconut rum
- 4 oz strawberry lemonade
- Ice cubes
- Fresh strawberry

Instructions:

1. Fill a glass with ice cubes.
2. Pour in the coconut rum and strawberry lemonade.
3. Stir gently to combine.

To Serve:

Garnish with a fresh strawberry on the rim or skewered on a cocktail pick. Enjoy your refreshing Dunk Bunny with beach vibes in every sip!

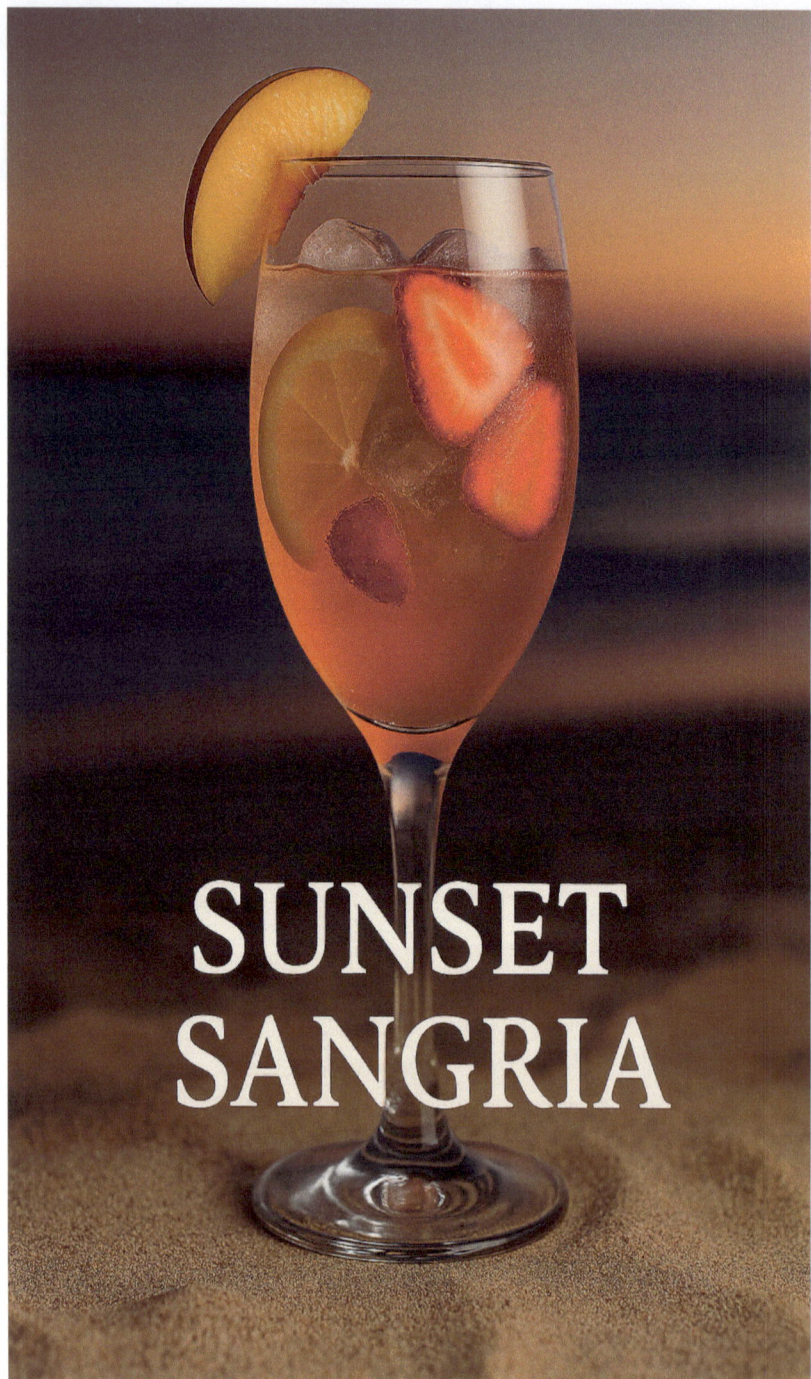

SUNSET
SANGRIA

Sunset Sangria

Ingredients:

- White wine
- Peach slices
- Strawberries
- Pink lemonade
- Ice cubes

Method:

1. In a large pitcher, combine chilled white wine with pink lemonade.
2. Add fresh peach slices and strawberries.

To Serve:

Stir well and pour over ice in your favourite glass. Let the glow of the sunset match the warmth of your glass.

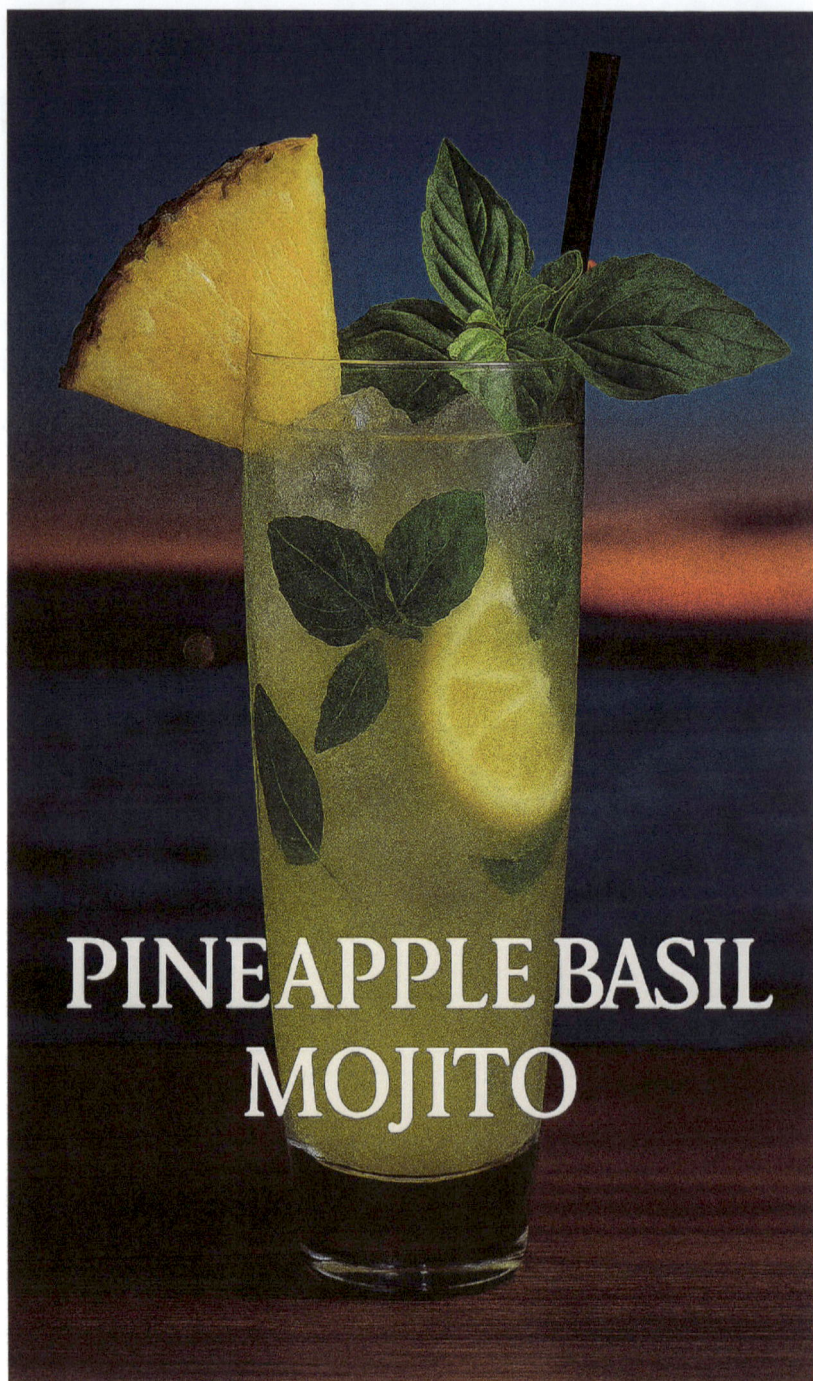

PINEAPPLE BASIL
MOJITO

Pineapple Basil Mojito

Ingredients:

- Crushed pineapple
- Fresh basil leaves
- Soda water
- Lime juice
- White rum (optional)

Method:

1. In a glass, muddle the crushed pineapple and basil leaves with a splash of lime juice.
2. Fill the glass with ice, then top with soda water.
3. Add white rum if desired for a refreshing kick.

To Serve:

Stir gently and garnish with a sprig of basil or a pineapple wedge. Sip, smile, and repeat!

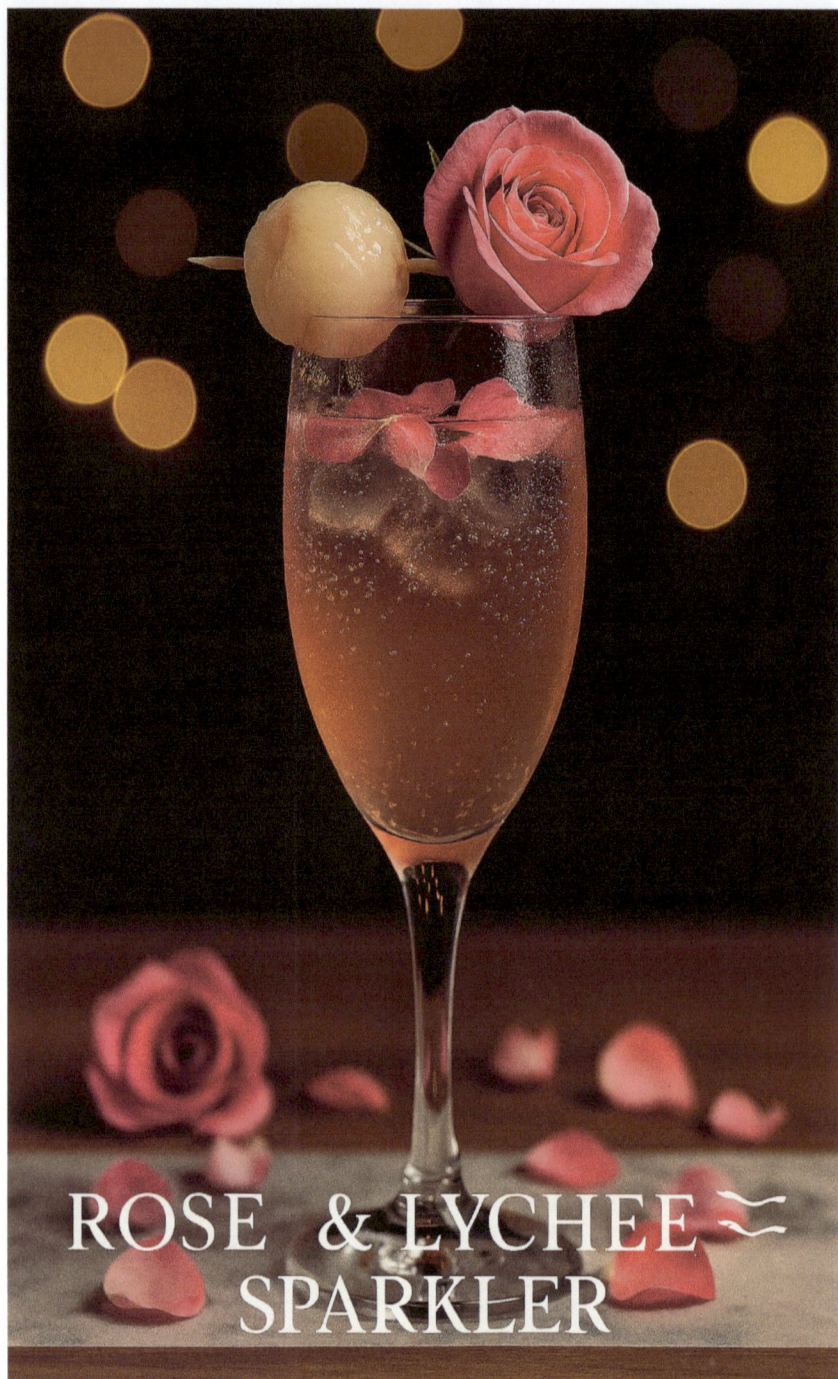

ROSE & LYCHEE SPARKLER

Rose & Lychee Sparkler

Ingredients:

- Lychee syrup
- Rose water
- Soda water
- Prosecco

Method:

1. In a chilled glass, combine a splash of lychee syrup with a dash of rose water.
2. Add a generous pour of soda water.
3. Top with prosecco for that perfect effervescent finish.

To Serve:

Garnish with a lychee or edible flower for a romantic touch. Best enjoyed at golden hour with your favourite playlist.

CITRUS CROWN COOLER

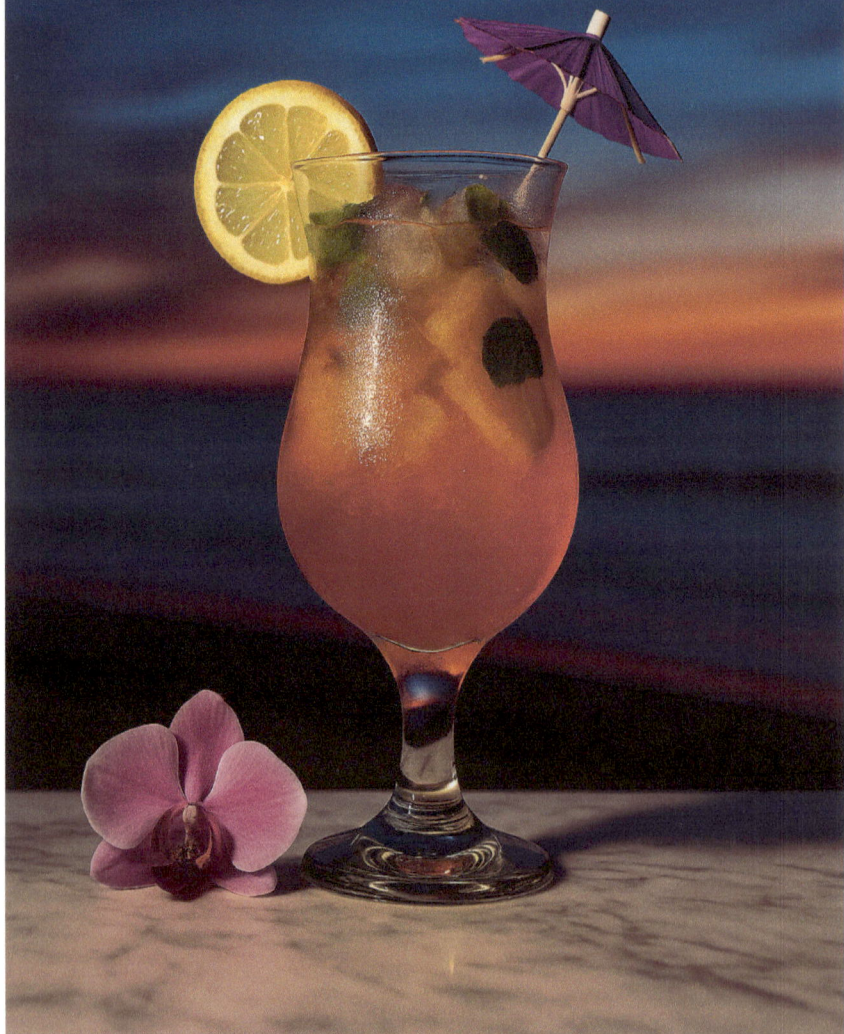

Citrus Crown Cooler

Ingredients:

- Grapefruit juice
- Lemon
- Passionfruit syrup
- Soda water
- Gin

Method:

1. In a shaker or mixing glass, combine grapefruit juice, a squeeze of fresh lemon, and passionfruit syrup.
2. Add a shot of gin and give it a good stir or light shake.
3. Pour over a tall glass filled with ice.
4. Top with soda water and garnish with a lemon slice or passionfruit pulp for extra flair.

To Serve:

Sip and reign over your refreshment realm.

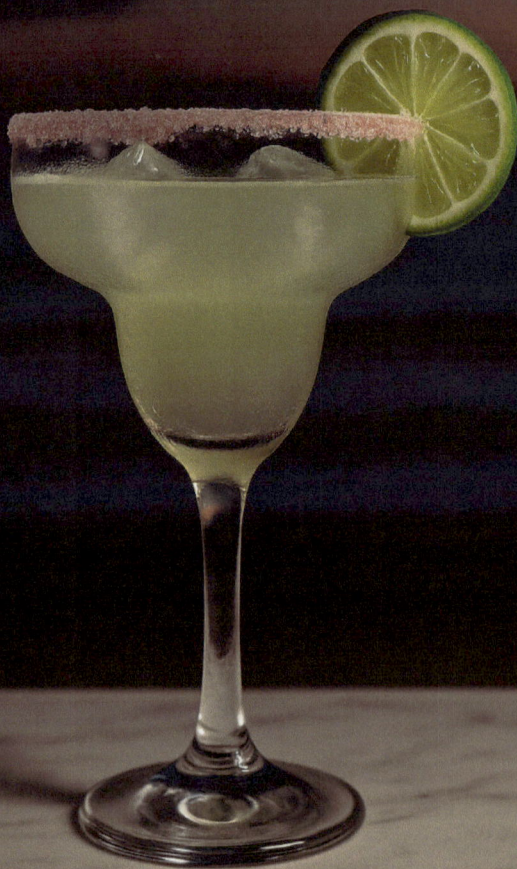

GLOW BAR
MOCKTAIL
MARGARITA

Mocktail Margarita

Ingredients:

- Coconut water
- Lime juice
- Agave
- Pink salt (for rim)
- Optional: Tequila

Method:

1. Moisten the rim of your glass with a lime wedge and dip it into pink salt to coat.
2. In a shaker, combine coconut water, lime juice, and agave. Add tequila if desired.
3. Shake with ice until chilled.

To Serve:

Strain into your prepared glass over fresh ice and enjoy your tropical refreshment!

Lavender Lemonade Spritz

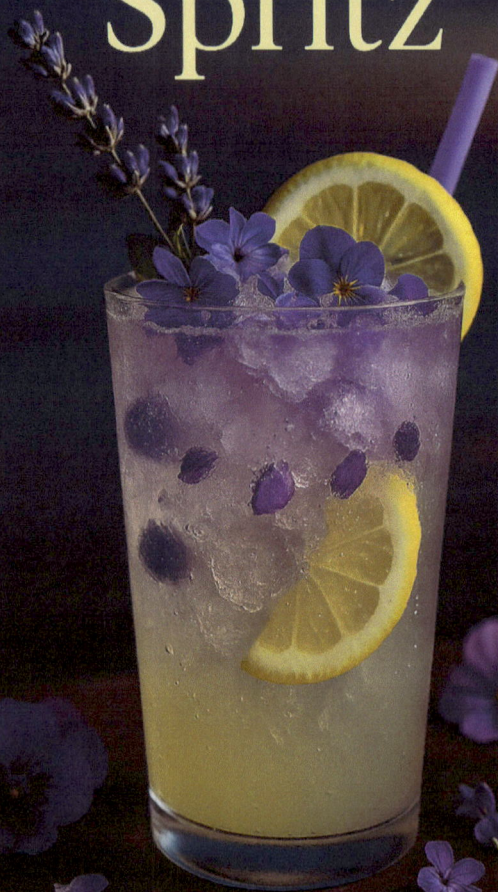

Lavender Lemonade Spritz

A delicate, floral refreshment that's as pretty as it is delicious.

Ingredients:

- Lavender syrup
- Lemonade
- Vodka (optional)
- Edible flowers

Method:

1. Fill a glass with ice and pour in lemonade and a splash of lavender syrup.
2. Add vodka if using.
3. Stir gently and top with edible flowers for an elegant finish.

To Serve:

Perfect for sunny afternoons or garden gatherings.

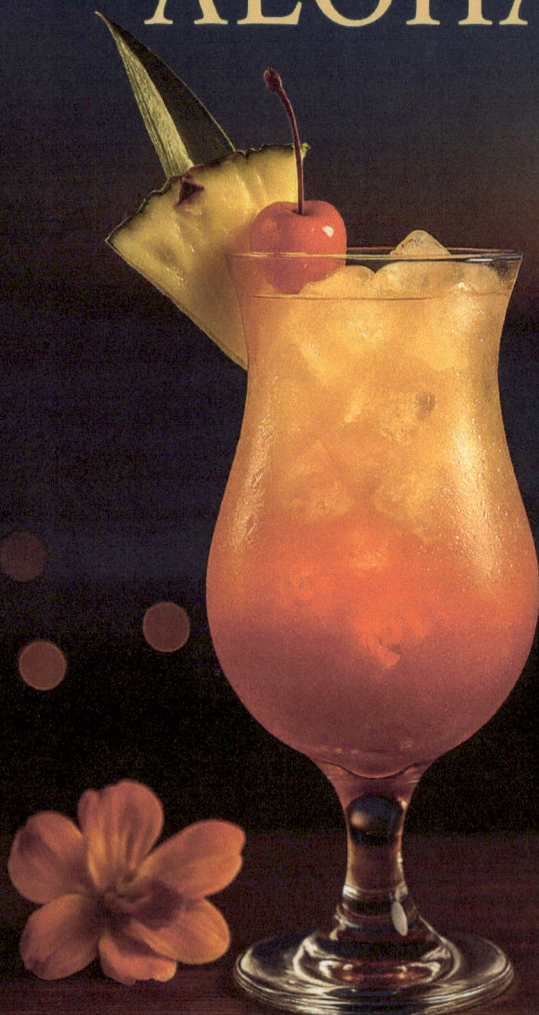

AMARETTO
ALOHA

AMARETTO ALOHA

Amaretto Aloha

Ingredients:

- Amaretto
- Pineapple juice
- Cranberry juice

Method:

1. Pour amaretto, pineapple juice, and cranberry juice over ice in a cocktail shaker.
2. Shake well until chilled.

To Serve:

Strain into a chilled glass and garnish with a pineapple wedge or cherry. Sip and feel the island breeze!